The Type 2
Diabetes
Handbook

Six Rules for Staying
Healthy with Type 2 Diabetes

Rod Colvin, M.S.
with James T. Lane, M.D.

Addicus Books, Inc.
Omaha, Nebraska

An Addicus Nonfiction Book

ISBN: 978-1-886039-64-3

Cover design by Jack Kusler
Illustrations by Jack Kusler
Typography by Linda Dageforde

This book is not intended to serve as a substitute for a physician. Nor is it the authors' intent to give medical advice contrary to that of an attending physician.

Library of Congress Cataloging in Publication

Colvin, Rod
    The type 2 diabetes handbook : six rules for staying healthy with type 2 diabetes / Rod Colvin ; with James T. Lane.
        p. cm.
    Includes index.
    ISBN 978-1-886039-64-3 (alk. paper)
1. Non-insulin-dependent diabetes—Popular works.
        I. Lane, James T. II. Title.
    RC660.4.C654 2011
    616.4'624—dc22   2010038447

Addicus Books, Inc.
P.O. Box 45327
Omaha, Nebraska 68145
www.AddicusBooks.com

Printed in the United States of America
10 9 8 7 6 5 4 3 2 1

Contents

Foreword

Type 2 diabetes is an epidemic in the United States. According to the American Diabetes Association, the number of cases of type 2 diabetes in the United States has almost quadrupled in the past thirty years—from 6 million cases in 1980 to 18 million today with an estimated 6 million who've not been diagnosed. The cost in terms of human suffering and healthcare dollars is staggering.

As an endocrinologist, I have treated diabetes patients for the past twenty years. I have seen the suffering this disease can bring. However, I also know that it is possible to prevent or significantly reduce this suffering. I work with other physicians, nurses, and diabetes educators to help patients understand type 2 diabetes so that they can avoid complications.

Diabetes is unlike other diseases in that you can make lifestyle changes to control it. As you'll read in this book, these changes involve eating right, losing weight, exercising, monitoring glucose levels, and taking medications as directed. This book will serve as a helpful tool for making your life healthier and happier.

James T. Lane, M.D., Medical Director
The Nebraska Medical Center
Diabetes Center

Acknowledgments

I would like to thank James T. Lane, M.D., Medical Director of the Nebraska Medical Center Diabetes Center, for serving as the medical editor for this book. His guidance and expertise were invaluable.

I also wish to thank members of Dr. Lane's staff for the expertise they shared, including Beth Pfeffer, Director of Diabetes Services, Lisa Nichter, dietician, and Kristina Volkmer, exercise physiologist.

I thank Karen Abrams, Anne Steinhoff, and Alyson Meadows for their research and editorial support. I express my appreciation to Jack Kusler, who provided the illustrations for the book.

To wish to be well is part of becoming well.
—Senca, Roman Philosopher

Rule 1

Learn the Basics about Type 2 Diabetes

Type 2 diabetes is an epidemic in the United States. The American Diabetes Association estimates 18 million Americans have been diagnosed with the disease and another 6 million others have it, but have not been diagnosed.

Type 2 diabetes develops most often in adults over the age of forty, but can develop in young people, too. If not kept under control, diabetes can cause serious complications. People with type 2 diabetes are two to three times more likely to have a heart attack or stroke. Diabetes is also the most common cause of kidney failure and blindness in adults under age sixty. Other potential complications include nerve damage, which may lead to pain and numbness in the hands and feet, and damage to blood vessels, which may result in amputation of limbs. Nerve damage can also affect many other bodily functions.

Coping Emotionally

It's never easy to hear from your doctor that you have a chronic disease such as type 2 diabetes. It's not uncommon to feel depressed after being told you have diabetes, and depression may have a negative effect on your health. When you're depressed, you may not feel motivated to take the best care of yourself. Consequently, you may not eat right or take medications as directed. These actions can cause blood sugars to rise even higher.

If you're like many people, you may at first go into denial about having type 2 diabetes. You may tell yourself things such as "This can't happen to me" or "My case will be different—I won't have problems like some other people do. After all, I don't really feel sick."

Denial is a common response to a diagnosis of diabetes. Perhaps initial denial allows our minds to accept the news more gradually. However, ongoing denial is a dangerous thing. It will prevent you from getting the care you need to manage the disease. Some people deny having the disease for years before taking action to control it; this lack of action over time significantly increases the risks for complications.

One way to break through denial is to talk with people you trust about having type 2 diabetes. Keeping it a secret feeds the denial. Discuss your thoughts and feelings openly. If you feel you would benefit from more emotional support, consider finding a therapist, a certified diabetes educator, or a support group. Once you accept the diagnosis, you'll be better prepared to start a treatment plan.

Defining Type 2 Diabetes

Type 2 diabetes is a metabolic disorder caused by the combination of the body's resistance to the effect of insulin (not using its own insulin efficiently) and the pancreas not producing enough insulin. As a result, there is an increase in the level of sugar, also known as glucose, in the blood. This causes a condition known as *insulin resistance*, which is at the root of type 2 diabetes. If you learn that you have high blood sugars, you may have been gradually becoming insulin resistant for several years.

In order to understand the concept of insulin resistance, let's review briefly how our food is digested and turned into energy. When food enters your body, it is broken down into small components, including *glucose*, an important sugar that comes from carbohydrates. Glucose is a major source of energy for the body. When you eat carbohydrates, your body detects a

2

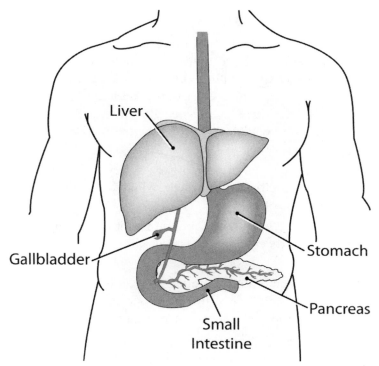

The pancreas is located behind the lower part of the stomach. Beta cells within the pancreas secrete insulin, which helps control carbohydrate metabolism.

rise in glucose and signals the pancreas to produce insulin. Together, glucose and insulin enter the bloodstream. The insulin allows the glucose to enter the cells of the muscles and liver to be used for energy.

If your body is not producing enough insulin, or if your body is not using the insulin efficiently, the glucose doesn't reach the cells. This causes a rise in glucose. Your body will counter with increased insulin production and secretion, which also causes an increase in the levels of insulin in the blood. There are multiple causes of insulin resistance.

Causes of Insulin Resistance

Obesity. Many people become insulin resistant when they are 35 to 40 percent above their ideal body weight. The extra weight overloads tissues with excess fatty acids in the blood and promotes insulin resistance. Obesity is a leading cause of insulin resistance. Nearly three-fourths of the people with type 2 diabetes are overweight; however, thin people, especially the elderly, can also develop diabetes.

Genetics. Your family history is a key factor in insulin levels. Genetics help to determine whether or not you will develop insulin resistance.

Physical inactivity. When muscle is not used regularly, it is less efficient at receiving and using glucose in response to insulin.

Stress. When the body is under stress, it releases a hormone called *cortisol.* Too much of this hormone is thought to play a role in the development of insulin resistance. Cortisol can also stimulate appetite and weight gain.

Infection or illness. An illness or infection raises the level of stress hormones critical for the body's ability to recover from the illness. The stress hormones actually work against the effect of insulin and cause further insulin resistance. In addition, high blood sugars inhibit the ability of the white blood cells to kill bacteria and may result in a greater risk of infection.

Pregnancy. The fluctuation of hormones during pregnancy may increase insulin resistance. For those women with an increased risk of type 2 diabetes later on, blood sugars may rise during pregnancy and result in a form of diabetes called *gestational diabetes.*

Ethnicity. The chances of having insulin resistance and being diagnosed with type 2 diabetes increase if your heritage is African American, American Indian, Alaska Native, Hispanic/Latino, Asian, or Pacific Islander.

Symptoms of Diabetes

The symptoms of diabetes may develop so gradually that you don't readily notice them. Many people have diabetes for several years before it's diagnosed. You may have some of the symptoms of type 2 diabetes, but you may not have all of them. The following list describes symptoms and why they occur.

Frequent urination and excessive thirst. When blood is filtered into the kidneys and blood sugars are high, you start excreting glucose into your urine. This causes the urine to pull more water out of your blood. As a result, you need to urinate more frequently. Frequent urination can cause dehydration, prompting you to feel excessive thirst.

Fatigue. When your body is not delivering glucose to the cells efficiently, your body is experiencing a form of starvation. It cannot use the energy from the food you eat. Energy production by many of the tissues in the body goes down. Consequently, you feel tired and lack energy.

Excessive hunger. When the body's cells are not receiving the glucose they need for energy, it can produce the sensation of hunger. The cells send a message to the brain that they need glucose; the brain interprets this signal as hunger.

Occasional blurry vision. When blood sugars are high, the glucose draws excess fluid into the eyeballs. This expansion of volume changes the focal point on the eye, causing occasional blurry vision.

Weight loss. This may not seem like a likely symptom since most people with type 2 diabetes are overweight. However, when your body does not use insulin adequately, body tissues, including muscle and fat, can break down as your body looks for alternative sources of fuel. Calories are excreted in the urine, and you experience a weight loss.

Sores or wounds that heal slowly. When you have a wound, the body uses proteins to repair tissues. When you have high blood sugars, your body does not produce structurally normal proteins. This slows healing.

Infections. With type 2 diabetes, you may have more infections than usual. Just as a high level of glucose affects other components in the blood, it also affects the white blood cells, which fight infection. Consequently, the white blood cells do not stave off infections normally.

Types of Diabetes

Diabetes mellitus is a metabolic disease characterized by high blood sugar levels, which result from defects in insulin response and secretion. In the United States, it is the seventh leading cause of death.

Type 1 diabetes usually develops during childhood or adolescence and occurs when the pancreas does not produce any insulin. However, it can also occur in adults. Those with type 1 diabetes must take insulin injections. About 10 percent of those with diabetes have type 1.

Type 2 diabetes is the result of the body not producing enough insulin or the body's cells ignoring the insulin. Type 2 diabetes can develop in youth as well as in adults. It affects about 90 percent of those with diabetes.

Gestational diabetes occurs in pregnant woman who have not previously had diabetes but whose blood sugars become elevated during pregnancy and return to normal after the pregnancy is over. Placental hormones make the mother resistant to insulin, causing a buildup of blood sugars. These women are at high risk for type 2 diabetes later on in their life.

Numbness or tingling sensations in the feet or hands. High glucose levels can damage nerves. Since the nerves in the feet and hands are the longest nerves in the body, they are the ones most commonly affected. You may experience a sensation of tingling or numbness.

Tests for Diagnosing Diabetes

The most commonly used test to diagnose type 2 diabetes is the *fasting blood glucose test.* Two other tests may also be used; they are the *random plasma glucose test* and the *oral glucose tolerance test.*

Fasting Blood Glucose Test

The fasting blood glucose test is the screening test favored by the American Diabetes Association. For this test, you must fast for six to eight hours. Then, blood is drawn from a vein in your arm and your blood sugar levels are tested.

If the test shows that you have a fasting blood sugar level above 126 mg/dl, you are usually diagnosed with type 2 diabetes. However, your doctor will likely perform the test a second time on another day to confirm the diagnosis.

Fasting Blood Glucose Classifications

Normal:	less than 100 mg/dl
Impaired fasting glucose:	100 to 125 mg/dl
Diabetes:	greater than 126 mg/dl

An impaired fasting glucose level means that your blood sugars are high, but not high enough to be classified as type 2 diabetes.

You will notice that the standard medical measurement used in blood tests is listed as "mg/dl," which refers to "milligrams per deciliter." A deciliter is one-tenth of a liter—a little less than half a cup. The body contains about 5.6 liters (six quarts), of blood.

Random Plasma Glucose Test

This test can be performed at any time without fasting. Blood is drawn and tested. For this test, a normal blood sugar level is below 140 mg/dl. If your test results are 200 mg/dl or above, and you have symptoms of diabetes, you can be diagnosed with type 2 diabetes.

Oral Glucose Tolerance Test

Although the oral glucose tolerance test is considered the most sensitive test for diagnosing type 2 diabetes, it's not considered the most convenient by patients. It takes longer than other tests and blood is drawn several times. For this test, you are asked to fast overnight, and a sample of your blood is drawn. Then, you are asked to drink a cup of liquid glucose. After drinking the glucose, your blood is drawn and tested again at two hours.

If you don't have type 2 diabetes, the blood glucose will rise and then return to normal because adequate insulin is produced in response to the sugary drink. However, if you do have diabetes, the blood glucose will rise higher than normal and come down at a much slower rate because not enough insulin is produced or the cells of the muscles and liver are not properly responding to the insulin.

If your oral glucose tolerance test result is 110 mg/dl or less, you have a normal glucose response and do not have diabetes. Your body is handling sugars normally.

If, at the two-hour mark during the test, your blood glucose is 140 mg/dl or higher but less than 200 mg/dl, you have *impaired glucose tolerance*. This means you are not processing glucose normally and are at increased risk for type 2 diabetes. If your blood glucose level at two hours is 200 mg/dl or greater, you will be diagnosed with type 2 diabetes.

Hemoglobin A1c Test

The *Hemoglobin A1c test* is another important means for measuring sugar levels in the blood. This test is different from others in that it tells what the blood sugar levels have been on average over a three-month period.

How is this test able to produce such a result? Hemoglobin A1c is a protein in red blood cells that bonds with blood sugars. Since red blood cells can live from 90 to 120 days, the hemoglobin A1c stays in the blood for that length of time. Accordingly, it is effective in measuring blood sugars over a period of time.

According to the American Diabetes Association, a normal A1c level is between 4 and 6 percent. A person with a level of 6.5 percent or higher is considered to have type 2 diabetes. This test is also used to assess blood sugar control as part of an ongoing monitoring strategy.

Disorders that Affect Type 2 Diabetes

As mentioned earlier, type 2 diabetes is a metabolic disorder. Other metabolic disorders, including abnormal blood fat (cholesterol and triglycerides) levels and high blood pressure, can be aggravated by type 2 diabetes. Similarly, high blood sugar levels can have a negative affect on cholesterol levels and blood pressure. In fact, if you a have a cluster of these metabolic disorders, you may have a condition known as *metabolic syndrome*.

Metabolic syndrome has also been called *Syndrome X* and *insulin resistance syndrome*. It's important to be aware of the disorders that make up this syndrome since they can affect your overall health. If you have metabolic syndrome, your risk of heart attack and stroke increases significantly. You are considered to have metabolic syndrome if you have three or more of the syndrome's five criteria.

1. *High fasting blood glucose.* This means blood glucose levels are higher than 110 (mg/dl) when tested after fasting, but are not yet high enough to be classified as diabetes.

2. *Abdominal obesity.* The fat around the belly, or "central obesity," is a key risk factor because it affects the body's metabolism. Men have central obesity if they have a waist circumference of 40 inches; for women, it is 35 inches.

3. *Low HDL cholesterol.* The high-density lipoprotein cholesterol (HDL) is known as the "good" cholesterol. For men, HDL levels of less than 45 mg/dl fit the criteria for metabolic syndrome; for women, the criteria is an HDL level of less than 55 mg/dl.

4. *High triglycerides.* Triglycerides are a form of fat the body uses for energy. Levels of more than 150 mg/dl are considered high for both men and women.

5. *High blood pressure.* High blood pressure, or hypertension, occurs when the force of blood flowing through the artery walls is too high. A blood pressure of 130/80 or more is considered high.

We've already discussed fasting blood glucose, so let's take a closer look at the other disorders in metabolic syndrome.

Abdominal Obesity

Medical experts believe that belly fat releases fatty acids and other hormones into the bloodstream, causing an increase in insulin resistance. It's also believed that abdominal fat cells produce toxic chemicals that disrupt the normal production of insulin and may promote chronic inflammation of tissues and the lining of blood vessels. These actions may also increase insulin resistance, which may promote high blood pressure and abnormal cholesterol levels.

Low HDL Cholesterol

Cholesterol is carried through the bloodstream by proteins. High-density lipoproteins, HDL, the "good cholesterol," acts as a scavenger in the bloodstream, carrying away harmful cholesterol to the liver for excretion from the body. This helps prevent the formation of clogged arteries, a condition known as *atherosclerosis.* When HDL cholesterol levels are too low, the good cholesterol is not able to function normally, and contributes to atherosclerosis, the buildup of cholesterol in the arteries.

HDL (Good) Cholesterol Levels

For women: 55 mg/dl or greater
For men: 45 mg/dl or greater

Low HDL cholesterol can be caused by a variety of factors, which include: high blood sugars, being overweight, lack of physical activity, cigarette smoking, high triglycerides, genetics, and some medications such as anabolic steroids.

High Triglycerides

Most of the stored fat in your body is made up of triglycerides. They come from fats in the food we eat; the body makes them from carbohydrates. When we eat, the calories we don't need immediately for energy are converted to triglycerides and transported to fat cells to be stored.

When the body needs energy, the fat tissue breaks down the triglycerides and releases them into the bloodstream as fatty acids. If you are overweight, too much fatty acid is released, and tissues become overloaded with fat. This contributes to insulin resistance and to the development of cardiovascular disease.

Triglyceride Levels

Normal:	less than 150 mg/dl
High:	250 mg/dl
Very high:	500 mg/dl

High triglycerides are caused by inactivity, a diet high in carbohydrates, cigarette smoking, excess consumption of alcohol, or a genetic tendency to metabolize fats abnormally.

High Blood Pressure

Blood pressure refers to the force on the artery walls as the heart pumps blood. It's measured in two forms. The pressure when the heart beats is called the *systolic pressure*; the pressure when the heart is at rest is the *diastolic pressure*. When your blood pressure is taken, it is expressed as the systolic pressure, which is higher, over the diastolic pressure, which is lower. For example, normal blood pressure is 120/80 or lower.

Although high blood pressure does not cause type 2 diabetes, insulin resistance is known to cause retention in the amount of sodium, or salt, in the bloodstream. This can increase the volume of blood circulating in the vessels, causing an increase in blood pressure. High blood pressure, also called *hypertension*, puts extra stress on the heart and can cause a heart attack or stroke. It can also put extra stress on the small blood vessels that are associated with eye and kidney damage in those with type 2 diabetes.

Blood Pressure Levels

	Systolic	Diastolic
Normal	120	Below 80
Pre-hypertension	120-139	80-89
Stage 1 hypertension	140-159	90-99
Stage 2 hypertension	160 or higher	100 or higher

The American Diabetes Association recommends having a blood pressure reading of less than 130/80.

High LDL Cholesterol

What's commonly called LDL cholesterol, the "bad" cholesterol, is not part of the criteria for metabolic syndrome; however, high levels of LDL (low-density lipoprotein) cholesterol are serious risk factors for heart attack and stroke. When you have too much LDL cholesterol in your bloodstream, the fats can build up and clog arteries, adding another risk to an already serious list of risk factors.

LDL (Bad) Cholesterol Levels

Normal:	70-100 mg/dl
High:	130-160 mg/dl
Very high:	greater than 160 mg/dl

High levels of LDL cholesterol can be caused by eating foods that are high in *saturated fats*. These types of fats come from animal sources and include such foods as egg yolks, cheese, and meats. Other factors that contribute to high LDL cholesterol levels include being overweight, lack of exercise, aging, and heredity (many people with elevated LDL cholesterol levels have an inherited tendency toward the increased levels).

Is Type 2 Diabetes Reversible?

Type 2 is not considered curable; however, making the right lifestyle changes will cause glucose levels to drop.

Numerous studies have shown that people with type 2 diabetes can reduce glucose levels to normal ranges by losing weight and exercising regularly. Some people are able to discontinue diabetes medications when blood sugar levels become normal.

Rules for Successfully Managing Type 2 Diabetes

Many chronic diseases progress regardless of the actions you take to combat them. However, type 2 diabetes is different from many other diseases—you can exert a great deal of control over the disease and stay healthy.

We are a "pill society"—we tend to think of treating any disease by taking a pill and being done with it. And yes, there are many medications available today that are effective in the treatment of type 2 diabetes, but medications are only part of a good care plan. There are six basic rules that will help you successfully manage type 2 diabetes. They are:

1. Learn the basics about type 2 diabetes.
2. Eat right and control your weight.
3. Exercise regularly.
4. Monitor blood sugar levels regularly.
5. Take medications as directed.
6. Avoid complications by practicing good self-care.

You'll learn more about these rules in the chapters that follow. The rules themselves are simple. Of course, the challenge is putting the rules into action. You'll be better prepared to take action if you take the crucial first step—educating yourself about type 2 diabetes.

You don't have to let diabetes control your life. You can take control of it.

Rule 2

Eat Right and Control Your Weight

The combination of eating a well-balanced diet and losing excess weight are two of the most important actions you can take to manage your diabetes. If you control what you eat, you can keep tight controls on your blood glucose level and prevent complications.

Managing your type 2 diabetes is not about going on a diet, but about developing good eating habits that you will be able to maintain over your lifetime. Making major changes in the way you've been eating can be challenging, but change will be easier if you start with a plan that helps you achieve small but important goals, one step at a time.

Setting those goals will be easier if you understand the basics of good nutrition.

Guidelines for Good Nutrition

Given all the food choices available today and the ease with which we can get food, it's important to understand the basics of balanced nutrition and maintaining a healthy weight. According to the American Diabetes Association, there are four basic tips that you can follow to ensure good nutrition and a healthy weight:

1. Eat a wide variety of foods every day.
2. Eat high-fiber foods, such as fruits, vegetables, whole grains, and beans.

3. Use less added fat and sugar, and reduce sodium intake (including table salt).
4. Be physically active every day.

Benefits of a Balanced Diet

There are many benefits to eating healthful foods. If you eat well, you'll not only feel better, but you'll enjoy better health in the long term. Here are other benefits of good nutrition if you're living with type 2 diabetes:

Maintains blood glucose levels. It's important to keep in mind that the main goal of blood sugar control is to bring your blood sugars down to healthy levels. Your healthcare provider will work with you to determine that level. A balanced eating plan will help you bring your blood sugars down.

It helps if you eat regularly. Basically, that means eating three regular meals a day, spaced evenly apart, along with healthful snacks in between. Also, work on developing a meal plan that helps you to balance your carbohydrate intake from one day to the next. Together, these steps will help you keep your blood glucose levels stable.

Maintains a healthy weight. A well-balanced, nutritious diet will help you attain a healthy weight. As explained earlier, being overweight interferes with your body's ability to properly use insulin. Being overweight increases the risk of developing other health concerns, including joint problems, gallbladder disease, colon and breast cancer, and breathing problems.

Lowers risks of cardiovascular complications. Eating the right foods means reducing your intake of saturated fat and keeping your cholesterol within a normal range. When your cholesterol levels are high, you are at risk for heart attack and stroke. With improved nutrition, your heart and arteries will be healthier and you will reduce your chances of cardiovascular disease.

Food Basics

Good nutrition involves eating a balanced diet of carbohydrates, protein, and good fats. If you understand the basics of these critical nutrients, and how to incorporate them into your diet, you will be well on the road to improving your eating habits.

Carbohydrates

Our bodies need energy to function. Glucose from carbohydrates is the body's main source of energy. Carbohydrates are made of starches and sugars, which all break down into glucose—the most simple sugar molecule—during digestion. It is the glucose level in the blood that we call your "blood sugar" level. Because your blood sugar levels are directly tied to the amount of carbohydrates you eat, understanding carbs is very important in managing your type 2 diabetes. Carbohydrates are divided into six core groups:

- grains and food made with grain
- beans
- starchy vegetables
- milk and yogurt
- fruit and fruit juices
- sweets and desserts

There is an additional category of carbohydrates, called "free" foods, because you can eat several servings of these a day without affecting your blood sugars. These free foods are primarily the nonstarchy vegetables, but also include artificial sweeteners and condiments such as ketchup and mustard, which we use in very small quantities.

For people with type 2 diabetes, it may seem that carbohydrates are the "enemy." However, it's important to remember that carbohydrates are an important part of a healthful diet. Instead of trying to cut carbs out of your diet entirely, try changing your goals to eat more-nutritious carbs.

One serving of carbohydrate has about fifteen grams of carbohydrate. You should work with your healthcare provider to determine the appropriate number of servings of carbs for you to eat in one day. Here are examples of foods that count as one serving of carbohydrates:

- 1 slice of bread
- 1 small apple
- ½ banana
- 1 cup milk
- 1 small white or sweet potato
- 3 cups popcorn

Eat more nutritious carbohydrates. For example, eat more whole grains, fruits, and nonstarchy vegetables, rather than less nutritious carbs such as snack crackers and white bread. At the same time, remember that more nutritious carbs are still carbs, and so they will still raise your blood glucose levels. Be sure to control portions.

Even out your carbohydrate intake. Balance your carbohydrate intake daily. This means avoid eating large portions of food that contain carbs at one meal and then eating only a few carbs at the next meal. This will help you avoid dramatic swings in the number of carbohydrates you ingest, which will help prevent spikes in blood sugars. As you maintain more stable blood sugar levels over time, you will feel better and your health will improve.

Current nutritional guidelines suggest that most Americans should be getting more vegetables, fruits, and whole grains in their diets. All these foods are rich in nutrients and contain healthier carbohydrates. When you digest these foods, you unlock rich sources of vitamins and minerals that help protect the cells in your body and improve the way your organs function. You can work with a nutritionist to identify healthful sources of carbs for your meal plan.

Recommended Sources of Carbohydrates

- Whole grains and foods made of grain: pasta, rice, cereal, oatmeal, tabbouleh, bread and buns, tortillas, pretzels, crackers
- Beans: black, chickpea, kidney, lentils, lima, mung, pinto, navy
- Starchy vegetables: peas, corn, potato, winter squash
- Non-fat or low-fat milk and yogurt
- Fruit (including dried fruit) and fruit juices: apple, banana, orange, pears, raisins, prunes

Eat sufficient amounts of fiber. A form of carbohydrate, fiber, also called roughage, is an important part of a healthful diet. Nutritious foods such as fresh fruits, vegetables, oats and other grains, beans, nuts, and seeds are high in fiber. Fiber can help you manage your blood glucose levels, lower your risk of heart disease, and help you lose weight.

Foods high in fiber are digested more slowly and so reduce the rate at which your body releases sugars into your bloodstream. This helps keep blood sugars stabilized. Fiber also has other benefits. It helps lower your blood pressure and may help reduce your overall cholesterol. Fiber has no calories, but helps make you feel full. Most Americans eat less than half of the fiber they should be getting. The American Diabetes Association recommends that people with type 2 diabetes eat twenty-five to thirty-five grams of fiber per day.

Limit certain carbohydrates. Be selective in the carbohydrates you choose. When you eat low-nutrient carbohydrates—white bread, non-whole-grain pasta, white rice, packaged cereals, rice cakes, crackers, cookies, and cakes—you're missing the benefits you would get if you ate nutrient-rich foods. Remember that low-nutrient carbs are "empty" calories, often high in fat, and can contribute to weight gain. Think before you eat, and work to limit your intake of low-nutrient carbohydrates. Choose, instead, whole-grain products, fruit, nonfat or low-fat yogurt.

Protein

Protein is essential to build and repair tissues; it should be part of your diet every day. Because protein doesn't break down into glucose, it has less effect on your blood sugar levels than carbohydrates do. Protein can be found in both plant and animal food sources. The key to choosing more nutritious protein is to select proteins that are low in fat, and low in saturated fat in particular. If you eat red meat, select lean cuts in order to reduce the amount of saturated fat you consume.

Raw nuts and seeds are delicious and healthful sources of plant protein that are also high in fiber. Although they contain heart-healthy unsaturated fat and are generally low in saturated fat, nuts are high in calories so enjoy them in moderation. Milk, yogurt, cheese, and other dairy products are another source of protein, but these foods are high in saturated fat when they are made from whole milk. As long as you select nonfat or low-fat milk and cheese products, you will get the protein content without the saturated fat.

Recommended Sources of Protein

- Nonfat or low-fat milk products: milk, yogurt, cottage and other cheeses
- Low-fat soy milk
- Eggs
- Chicken and turkey: light meat without the skin
- Fish: sole, tuna (including canned tuna in water)
- Very lean cuts of beef
- Tofu and tempeh
- Nuts

Good Fats

We all need *some* fat as part of a nutritious diet. We can't live without it. Fats keep cell membranes fluid and flexible. They promote growth of cells, blood vessels, and nerves, and they keep skin and other tissues lubricated. However, not all fats are alike—some are better for you than others. The good fats are unsaturated fats.

19

Unsaturated fats are recommended because they help to reduce cardiovascular disease by lowering levels of the artery-clogging cholesterols. There are two types of unsaturated fats: *polyunsaturated fats* and *monounsaturated fats.*

Polyunsaturated fat is a nutrient that provides dietary energy without raising cholesterol levels. These fats are popular because of their health benefits—in particular, protecting against heart disease and stroke. Although these fats are necessary for our health, our bodies can't make them so we must get them from the foods we eat. They are found in foods such as corn oil, safflower-seed oil, sunflower-seed oil, and flaxseed oil.

The fats known as *omega-3 fatty acids* are also examples of polyunsaturated fats. They're found at particularly high levels in cold-water, fatty fish such as salmon, herring, sardines, tuna, trout, and mackerel. Other foods high in omega-3 fatty acids include ground flax-seeds and flaxseed oil, and walnuts. In order to ensure you get the omega-3 fatty acids you need, the American Diabetes Association recommends you eat two servings of fatty fish per week. Eat grilled or broiled fish, not fried.

> ### Recommended Sources of Fats
> *Polyunsaturated Fats*
> - Oils: safflower-seed, sunflower-seed, corn, sesame, flaxseed, soybean, fish
> - Fatty fish: salmon, tuna, mackerel, herring, trout, sardines
> - Nuts and seeds: walnuts, pine nuts, ground flaxseed, ground sesame seeds (tahini)
>
> *Monounsaturated Fats*
> - Oils: canola, olive, peanut, sesame
> - Avocado
> - Nuts and nut butter: peanuts, almonds, pecans, pistachios

Monounsaturated fat is another type of nutrient that provides dietary energy without raising cholesterol levels. These good fats are found in such foods as olive oil, canola oil, and peanut oil.

Bad Fats

Fats you should limit include saturated fats and trans fats. Both of these fats raise your levels of "bad" LDL cholesterol, increasing your risk of heart disease and stroke.

Saturated fats are found in animal sources such as meat, eggs, whole-milk products (including butter, cream, sour cream, cheese, cream cheese, cottage cheese, yogurt), and some plant foods, including coconut oil, palm fruit oil, and palm kernel oil. The American Diabetes Association recommends limiting saturated fat to 7 percent or less of your total calories each day.

Trans fats are fats that are artificially created through a chemical process called *hydrogenation*. This process solidifies the oils, which extends the shelf life of food products.

> ### Fats to Use Sparingly
> - Meat and meat products: beef, pork, poultry
> - Milk products: butter, cream, sour cream
> - Lard and shortening
> - Plant products: coconut oil and palm kernel oil

These hydrogenated fats are found in commercially prepared baked goods, margarine, snack foods, and processed foods. Commercially fried foods, such as french fries, are high in trans fats. These fats are considered to be the most harmful to one's health.

The main points to keep in mind for a healthful diet are: reduce your overall intake of fat, and when you do eat fat, choose healthful fats. And always remember that even good fats are high in calories.

Sodium

Sodium is an important consideration in your diet. Sodium is naturally present in many foods. It is also added to many prepared foods as a preservative or to add flavor. Be aware that many fast foods, canned goods, crackers, and other processed and prepared foods can be very high in sodium. Table salt, which we use with meals, is commonly a primary source of sodium in our diet.

21

People with type 2 diabetes are more sensitive to the effects of sodium, including the fact that sodium raises blood pressure. It's important, therefore, to keep your sodium intake low. Check food labels for the amount of sodium in each serving of prepared food. In addition, you should work with your healthcare provider to determine the specific amount of sodium that will be healthful for you to eat each day.

Alcohol

If you choose to drink alcohol, do so in moderation and with care. People with type 2 diabetes need to balance alcohol intake with meals and medication. It is critical for you to be aware of how alcohol will affect your blood sugars. The American Diabetes Association offers this advice:

- Check your blood glucose level before drinking because alcohol can cause hypoglycemia (low blood sugar).
- If you drink in the evening, check to make sure your blood glucose is at a safe level before bedtime, and eat something to raise it if it's not.
- Don't drink alcohol when your blood sugar is low.
- Don't drink on an empty stomach.
- Think before you drink—don't let the effects of alcohol interfere with your commitment to eating right.

Some people with type 2 diabetes shouldn't drink at all. For those who choose to drink, the American Diabetes Association recommends two drinks or less per day if you are a man, and one drink or less per day if you are a woman. One serving of alcohol is a regular or light 12-ounce beer, 5 ounces of wine, or 1.5 ounces of hard liquor.

If you take any medication, including diabetes medication, it is important that you check with your doctor about drug and alcohol interactions—some of these interactions can be dangerous. Also, keep in mind that if you are trying to lose weight, alcohol is high in calories. And when you add mixes for mixed drinks, you are adding both calories and carbs. Finally, if you have a history of alcohol abuse, or are pregnant, you should not drink alcohol at all.

Meal Plans

Your meal plan is a method for establishing a regular eating routine that identifies how much and what kinds of food to eat at each meal. Creating a meal plan is a disciplined approach to eating.

It's important to remember that creating a meal plan is *not* about what you can and cannot eat. Ultimately, it's really about portion control and moderation. For example, you still can have dessert, but your meal plan will help you stay smart about how much dessert you can have and how frequently.

There are many ways to create good meal plans. Working with a dietician will help you hone in on the meal plan that's best for you. Three common methods of meal planning are the ADA Create Your Plate method, the carb counting method, and the ADA Food Pyramid.

Create Your Plate

The Create Your Plate method, created by the ADA, was developed to give individuals with diabetes a fast, simple, and effective way to begin changing their eating habits in order to manage blood glucose levels. You start by cutting back on the overall amount of food you eat each day, and then graduate toward choosing healthier food to fill your plate. With this method, you eat the foods you want, but progress toward eating larger portions of nonstarchy vegetables and smaller portions of starchy foods and meat or other protein.

The following will help you create your plate for lunch and dinner:

1. Imagine a line down the middle of your dinner plate. Then imagine cutting one side in half so you now have three sections on your plate.

ADA's Create Your Plate

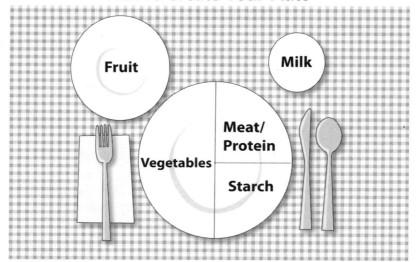

For the ADA's Create Your Plate meal plan, reserve half the plate for nonstarchy vegetables. The remaining sections are for meats and starchy foods. Servings of milk and fruit are also recommended.

2. Fill the largest section with nonstarchy vegetables such as:

   - spinach, carrots, lettuce, greens, cabbage, bok choy
   - green beans, broccoli, cauliflower, tomatoes
   - vegetable juice, salsa, onion, cucumber, beets, okra
   - mushrooms, peppers, turnip

3. In one of the small sections, place starchy foods such as:

   - whole-grain breads, such as whole wheat or rye
   - whole-grain, high-fiber cereal
   - cooked cereal such as oatmeal, grits, hominy, or cream of wheat
   - rice, pasta, or tortillas
   - cooked beans and peas, such as pinto beans or black-eyed peas

- potatoes, green peas, corn, lima beans, sweet potatoes, or winter squash
- low-fat crackers and snack chips, pretzels, or light popcorn

4. In the other small section, put your meat or meat substitutes such as:

- chicken or turkey without the skin
- fish such as tuna, salmon, cod, or catfish
- other seafood such as shrimp, clams, oysters, crab, or mussels
- lean cuts of beef and pork such as sirloin or pork loin
- tofu, eggs, or low-fat cheese

5. Add an 8-ounce glass of nonfat or low-fat milk. If you don't drink milk, you can add another small serving of carbs such as a 6-ounce container of light yogurt or a small roll.

6. Add a piece of fresh fruit or a half cup of fruit salad (fresh, frozen, or canned in juice or frozen in light syrup), and you have your meal planned.

For breakfast, follow the same idea. Use half the plate for starchy foods. Add fruit and meat in the remaining sections.

Carb Counting

The carb counting method is an accurate way of keeping track of the number of carbohydrates you eat throughout the day and adjusting your carbohydrate intake based on your blood glucose levels. Carb counting requires you to be quite diligent in monitoring your blood glucose levels and in tracking your carbohydrate intake.

To do carb counting properly, you will need to use a scale, measuring cups, and measuring spoons to consistently measure the grams of carbohydrates you eat in each serving. After a couple of weeks, you will find that you have developed a knack for accurately determining serving sizes of foods containing carbs without measuring. You will also need to understand food labels.

There are many resources available to help you accurately count carbs. Ask your doctor or dietician for assistance accessing these resources. To see examples of daily meal plans that show counts for both carbs and calories, see the Appendix in the back of this book.

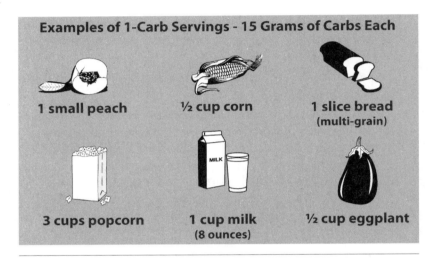

Examples of 1-Carb Servings - 15 Grams of Carbs Each

1 small peach   **½ cup corn**   **1 slice bread** (multi-grain)

3 cups popcorn   **1 cup milk** (8 ounces)   **½ cup eggplant**

Carb Counting Food List

Fifteen grams is one serving of carbs.

Breads: 15g Carbs
1 slice bread
6 small breadsticks (4" long)
½ English muffin, hot dog or
    hamburger bun
1 small croissant
1 matzo ball
1 small muffin* (1 oz.)
1 5" pancake/waffle*
½ pita (6")
1 small plain roll (1 oz.)
1 slice fruit bread (¼" thick)

1 tortilla (6")
⅓ c stuffing*
2"x 2" cornbread or biscuit

Cereal: 15g Carbs
½ c bran cereal
¼ c granola*
½ c cooked cereal
¾ c dry cereals
½ c sugar frosted cereal
1 ½ c puffed cereal

26

Crackers/snack food: 15g Carbs
6-7 animal crackers
3 graham crackers
3 c light popcorn
4-6 round crackers*
¾ oz. pretzels (15 mini twists)
1 oz. snack chips* (10-15)
6 saltine crackers

Pasta/grains: 15g Carbs
½ c chow mein noodles*
$\frac{1}{3}$ c pasta, other grains (cooked)
$\frac{1}{3}$ c brown/white rice (cooked)
½ c fried rice*

Milk/yogurt: 15g Carbs
1 c skim, 2%, whole, buttermilk*
½ c evaporated skim milk
$\frac{1}{3}$ c nonfat dry milk powder
1 c plain yogurt
¾ -1 c artificially sweetened yogurt

Combination Foods: 30g Carbs
1 c beef stew*
1 meat burrito*
2 stuffed cannelloni*
12 chicken nuggets
1.5 c chili w/beans*
1 small beef enchilada
1 3"x 4" piece lasagna*
2/3 c macaroni & cheese*
   or pasta salad*
1 pot pie* (7 oz.)
1 c ravioli*
2 soft-shell tacos*
1 tostada w/beans*
1 c casserole/hot dish
6 breaded fish sticks
¼ c ketchup
1 slice frozen pizza thick crust
2 slices frozen pizza thin crust
½ c tomato/marinara canned sauce

Potatoes/vegetables/beans: 15g Carbs
$\frac{1}{3}$ c beans (kidney, pinto) cooked
¼ c baked beans (canned)
½ c corn, hominy, peas
1 small white or sweet potato (3 oz.)
10-15 french fries*
½ c hash browns, au gratin*
1 c winter squash
1 c marinara or pasta sauce
½ c mashed potatoes

Fruits: 15g Carbs
1 small apple, orange, tangerine,
   pear, peach
½ c applesauce (unsweetened)
4 apricots (medium, fresh)
7 apricot halves (dried)
½ banana
2 T dried fruit
1 c cantaloupe
1 c melon cubes (cantaloupe,
   watermelon, or honeydew)
½ c cherries
2 figs, plums
½ c canned fruit (unsweetened)
½ grapefruit
15 grapes
½ c juice (unsweetened;
   grapefruit/orange)
1 large kiwi
¾ c pineapple, fresh
½ mango, papaya
3 medium prunes
2 T raisins or craisins
1 c strawberries/
   blueberries/raspberries

27

Vegetables: 5g Carbs
½ c cooked vegetables (asparagus, green beans, bean sprouts, broccoli, cabbage, carrots, cauliflower, eggplant, spinach, tomato, turnips, water chestnuts, zucchini
1 c raw vegetable
½ c tomato/vegetable juice
¼ c tomato puree

Soups: 15g Carbs
1 c broth base (chicken/beef noodle)
½ c bean, split pea
1 c cream soup*

Sweets: 15g Carbs
2" brownie (unfrosted)
2" square piece of cake (no icing)
2 small fat-free cookies
½ c custard
$\frac{1}{3}$ c frozen fat-free fruit yogurt
1 small granola bar*
½ c ice cream* or ice milk

½ twin popsicle or 1 fudgesicle
½ c sugar-free pudding
5 vanilla wafers
2 T light maple syrup
1 T all fruit jelly/jam
1 3" cookie

Sweets: 30g Carbs
2" square piece of cake w/icing
frosted cupcake *
$\frac{1}{8}$ pumpkin or custard pie*
½ c regular pudding*
1 c chocolate milk*
small soft serve cone*
½ large bagel (2 oz.)

Sweets: 45g Carbs
$\frac{1}{6}$ pc 2-crust pie*
$\frac{1}{6}$ pc Stir N' Frost carrot cake*
$\frac{1}{6}$ pc chocolate cheese cake*
1 small sweet roll or Danish*
1 c low fat yogurt w/fruit
2 T regular maple syrup

*Contains fat
Reprinted with permission from the Nebraska Medical Center Diabetes Center.

The ADA Food Pyramid

The ADA's Food Pyramid is a good guide for determining how many servings of each type of food you should eat each day. The pyramid, developed for people with diabetes, groups foods based on their carbohydrate and protein content. It provides a good model for eating a variety of foods every day to get all the nutrients and vitamins you need.

The foods at the top of the pyramid are those the ADA recommends eating in smaller quantities, and foods at the top of the pyramid, in greater amounts. For example, the pyramid recommends that you eat more grains, whole-wheat breads, starchy vegetables, and fruits than anything else. Nonfat or low-fat milk and dairy products and lean meat and meat substitutes should be eaten in moderation. The pyramid also suggests that you eat far fewer fatty foods and sweets compared to food in the other categories.

The pyramid gives a range of servings. If you follow the minimum number of servings in each group, you would eat about 1,600 calories, and if you eat at the upper end of the range, it would be about 2,800 calories. Serving sizes for each food group is listed on page 30.

The ADA Food Pyramid

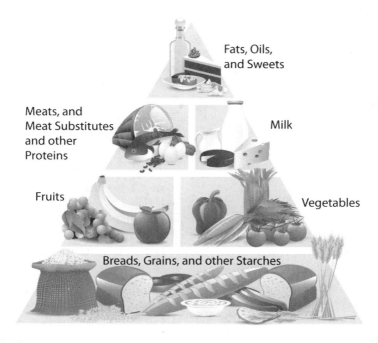

The ADA Food Pyramid recommends that food plans be made up of more of the foods at the bottom of the pyramid and fewer of the foods toward the top.

ADA Food Pyramid

Recommended Daily Servings

Grains: 6-11 servings
- 1 slice of bread
- ½ English muffin or hamburger bun
- ½ cup cooked cereal
- ¾ cup cooked cereal
- 1 tortilla (6-inch)
- ½ potato, yam, peas, corn, cooked beans
- $\frac{1}{3}$ cup rice or pasta

Vegetables: 3-5 servings
- spinach
- chicory
- sorrel
- Swiss chard
- broccoli
- cabbage
- bok choy
- brussels sprouts
- kale
- cauliflower
- carrots
- tomatoes
- cucumbers
- lettuce

Serving sizes: 1 cup raw or ½ cup cooked

Fruit: 2-4 servings
- blackberries
- cantaloupe
- strawberries
- oranges
- apples
- bananas
- peaches
- apricots
- grapes

Serving sizes: ½ cup canned fruit, 1 small fresh fruit, 2 T. dried fruit, 1 cup melon or raspberries, 1¼ cup whole strawberries

Meat, poultry, and fish: 4-6 oz.(total) per day
- beef
- chicken
- turkey
- fish
- eggs
- tofu
- dried beans
- cheese
- cottage cheese
- peanut butter

Serving sizes: Choose lean meats. Consume 4-6 oz. for the day. A serving size is 3 oz., about the size of a deck of cards.

Dairy: 2-3 servings
- 1 egg
- 1 cup milk
- 1 cup yogurt
- 1 ounce or ½ cup cheese
- ½ cup cottage cheese

Fats and sweets: use sparingly
- ½ cup ice cream
- 1 small cupcake or muffin
- 2 small cookies

Source: American Diabetes Association

Tips for Grocery Shopping

Your meal plan will help you control how and what you eat, and consequently it will help you control your blood sugars. When you are grocery shopping, there are things you can do that will help you choose the right foods to keep your diabetes in check.

Shop the perimeter of your grocery store. Around the edges of the store is where the fresh fruits and vegetables, fresh meats, and dairy products are usually located. You will notice that the middle aisles contain many more-refined and processed foods.

Don't go grocery shopping when you are hungry. The likelihood that you will make good food choices may be diminished if you go shopping when you are hungry. On the other hand, if you are full when you go grocery shopping, you are more likely to avoid buying unhealthful foods on impulse.

Choose healthful fruits and vegetables. One trick for selecting a variety of healthful fruits and vegetables is to select them by color. Deep, rich colors, such as deep green or deep red, are best. Some of the rainbow of fruits and vegetables you can choose from are:

- *Red:* tomatoes, watermelon, red cabbage, cranberries, red potatoes, raspberries, red grapes
- *Yellow and Orange:* carrots, butternut squash, mangoes, apricots, oranges, pumpkins, sweet potatoes
- *Green:* lettuce, spinach, peas, broccoli, cucumbers, cabbage, kiwis, limes
- *Blue and Purple:* blueberries, raisins, eggplants, purple grapes, blackberries
- *White:* bananas, cauliflower, garlic, jicamas, onions, turnips, potatoes

Learn to Read Food Labels

For you to shop for groceries wisely, it's important that you learn how to read and understand food labels. They will provide you with the information you need to maintain a nutritious diet.

Serving Size: All information on the label is based on this one cup serving size.

Total Fat: This gives the total grams of fat in a serving.

Saturated Fat/Trans Fat: These are grams of "bad" fats.

Total Carbohydrate: Label shows total grams of carbohydrates in one serving. Includes all starches, sugars, dietary fiber, and sugar alcohols.

Nutrition Facts

Serving Size 1 cup (228g)
Servings Per Container 2

Amount Per Serving	
Calories 260	Calories from Fat 120

	% Daily Value*
Total Fat 13g	**20%**
Saturated Fat 5g	**25%**
Trans Fat 2g	
Cholesterol 30mg	**10%**
Sodium 660mg	**28%**
Total Carbohydrate 31g	**10%**
Dietary Fiber 0g	**0%**
Sugars 5g	
Protein 5g	

Vitamin A 4%	•	Vitamin C 2%
Calcium 15%	•	Iron 4%

*Percent Daily Values are based on a 2,000 calorie diet.

Understanding food labels also helps make you a savvy shopper, which means you'll understand that food companies' goal is to sell their products, not to make you healthy.

Labels such as "sugar-free," "fat-free," and "dietetic" don't necessarily mean the food is the best alternative for you. For example, although "sugar-free" may mean no added sugar, it doesn't mean no carbohydrates. Any simple carbohydrate will quickly change to sugar once ingested. Become familiar with the following label information.

Serving size. The amount of the product the food manufacturer has identified as "one serving." You may be surprised to see that what is called "one serving" is often much less than you might usually eat. If you eat more than the amount listed as one serving, you will be eating more calories than are listed on the label, and the amount of fat, cholesterol, sodium, carbohydrates, and protein you ingest as a result will increase as well.

Calories. The number of calories in a single serving. The number of calories you actually eat will depend on the number of servings you actually eat.

Fat. The grams (g) of fat in a single serving. Under "total fat," the label lists the grams of saturated as well as trans fats. To maintain a healthful diet, it is best to limit both saturated fat and trans fats.

Cholesterol. The number of milligrams (mg) of cholesterol per serving. People with type 2 diabetes are at higher risk for heart disease, so it is important to take steps to limit dietary cholesterol.

Sodium. The number of milligrams (mg) of sodium in a serving. People with type 2 diabetes are at higher risk for high blood pressure and other cardiovascular problems. Consuming too much sodium contributes to high blood pressure. Try to reduce your sodium intake. Low-sodium products have less than 140 mg of sodium per serving.

Total carbohydrates. The number of grams (g) of carbohydrates per serving. Under "total carbohydrates," you will find the subcategories of "dietary fiber" and "sugars." (Note that both fiber and sugars count toward the "total carbohydrates" number.) Since carbohydrates turn into glucose after digestion, the number of total carbohydrates is an important number. If you are counting carbs for your meal plan, this total carbs number is the one to count. Fiber is also important, because as part of a nutritious diet you will likely want to increase your fiber intake.

Protein. The total number of grams of protein in a serving. Proteins are found in grains, milk, meat, beans, nuts, and seeds.

Percent (%) daily value. The percent daily value represents how much of the recommended daily amount of a nutrient you will get from a single serving. For example, if the "% daily value" for sodium is listed as 15%, it means one serving of the food item has 15% of the sodium you should be receiving each day. However, this calculation is based on an average consumption of 2,000 calories per day. The correct daily value for you will be based on the number of calories you should be eating. Check with your healthcare provider to determine your personal daily calories and values goals. Note that you won't see "% daily value" listed for trans fats because the Food and Drug Administration doesn't yet have enough research information to accurately assess that number.

Vitamins and minerals. Note that vitamins A and C, as well as calcium, thiamin, niacin, iron, and riboflavin, can be listed, among other vitamins and minerals, along with their "% daily value" per serving, at the very bottom of the food label.

Dining-Out Options

It's easy to relax your vigilance and lose control of your meal plan when you eat away from home. The following tips will help you stay on track at restaurants.

Control portions. Be aware that even standard serving sizes in restaurants are often quite large. Never select the "jumbo" choice. Other tips to help you maintain portion control include:

- Avoid the buffet. The "all-you-can-eat" buffet can be an invitation to lose control. If a buffet meal is your only option, try to fill up as much of your plate as possible with vegetables and salad.
- Share your meal.
- Take home a "doggy bag." If you have a tendency to eat everything on your plate, ask your server to wrap up half your portion immediately upon being served.

Choose the right restaurant. Choose restaurants with more healthful menus. Some restaurants list foods on their menus as being "heart healthy."

Substitute. Choose the side salad or vegetable instead of the french fries. Opt for an oil-and-vinegar salad dressing instead of the higher-calorie dressings. Drink water instead of alcohol or caloric sodas. Use mustard instead of mayonnaise.

Avoid extras. Avoid toppings such as bacon bits, grated cheese, and sour cream. When offered dressings and gravy, order them on the side and use them in moderation, or don't get them at all. If you do end up with an "extra," choose a low-fat option such as light margarine, light dressing, light sour cream, low-fat cheeses, and low-fat mayonnaise.

Limit fast food. Fast food is usually high in calories, fat, sodium, and carbohydrates; frequently comes in "supersize" portions; and often is low in nutritional value. If you find yourself at a fast-food restaurant, choose meat items that are grilled, and leave off the cheese and mayonnaise. Many fast-food restaurants offer salads with low-fat dressing or fruit. Choose a diet beverage or water instead of a sugary soda.

Eat smart. Choose entrees that are made with vegetables and whole grains. Cut excess fat and fatty skin off meat. Avoid fried foods—choose baked or grilled options instead. Choose to eat only one carbohydrate per meal. For example, you may have the option of bread, rice, or potatoes. Select just one.

If you have trouble sticking to your meal plan when you eat out, talk with a dietician about how to make wise food choices when dining out. Also, limit the number of times you allow yourself to eat out each month.

Eating at the Homes of Friends and Family

When eating at the home of a friend or family member, you can follow many of the same tips for dining out. One advantage of dining at friends' and family's homes is that you will probably feel comfortable enough to tell them that you are following a meal plan and need to eat certain foods in order to keep your type 2 diabetes in check.

Maintaining a Healthy Weight

As emphasized earlier, obesity is a major contributing factor for diabetes. Being overweight interferes with your body's ability to properly use insulin. Managing your weight will help you manage your type 2 diabetes. Studies show that losing only 5 to

10 percent of your body weight can have tremendous health benefits for people with type 2 diabetes. Work with your doctor or diabetes educator to set appropriate weight-loss goals. Develop a meal plan that helps you maintain stable blood sugar levels and also helps you lose weight.

Body Mass Index Table

BMI	Normal		Overweight					Obese			
	19	24	25	26	27	28	29	30	35	40	50
Height	Weight in Pounds										
4'10"	91	115	119	124	129	134	138	143	167	191	239
4'11"	94	119	124	128	133	138	143	148	173	198	247
5'0"	97	123	128	133	138	143	148	153	179	204	255
5'1"	100	127	132	137	143	148	153	158	185	211	264
5'2"	104	131	136	142	147	153	158	164	191	218	273
5'3"	107	135	141	146	152	158	163	169	197	225	282
5'4"	110	140	145	151	157	163	169	174	204	232	291
5'5"	114	144	150	156	162	168	174	180	210	240	300
5'6"	118	148	155	161	167	173	179	186	216	247	309
5'7"	121	153	159	166	172	178	185	191	223	255	319
5'8"	125	158	164	171	177	184	190	197	230	262	328
5'9"	128	162	169	176	182	189	196	203	236	270	338
5'10"	132	167	174	181	188	195	202	209	243	278	348
5'11"	136	172	179	186	193	200	208	215	250	286	358
6'0"	140	177	184	191	199	206	213	221	258	294	368
6'1"	144	182	189	197	204	212	219	227	265	302	378
6'2"	148	186	194	202	210	218	225	233	272	311	389
6'3"	152	192	200	208	216	224	232	240	279	319	399
6'4"	156	197	205	213	221	230	238	246	287	328	410

Source: National Institutes of Health

Body Mass Index

To assess the amount of body fat you have, your doctor will likely calculate your body mass index (BMI). It is a measurement of weight in relation to height for adults. Although the BMI does not determine your percentage of body fat, it is widely used as a diagnostic tool to identify weight categories that may lead to health problems. The BMI determines whether you are underweight, overweight, or obese.

To find your BMI, consult the BMI chart—look for your height and weight and look up the corresponding BMI. Your BMI may identify you as a candidate for a weight-loss drug; such drugs are often recommended for those with a BMI above 27.

Weight Loss Tips

Go slow. Set realistic goals. Avoid fad diets that promise a quick fix. There is no magic pill for weight loss. In fact, people who lose weight too quickly usually gain it back, sometimes adding even more pounds. One of the main problems with fad diets is that when you set too fast a pace for weight loss, you don't give yourself a chance to actually change your eating and lifestyle habits.

Control portions. Just as controlling how much food you put on your plate is important for controlling your carb intake,

Carbohydrate Servings for Weight Control

Men

To lose weight	2-3 servings (30-45 grams)
To maintain weight	4-5 servings (60-75 grams)
For active men	4-6 servings (60-90 grams)

Women

To lose weight	2-3 servings (30-45 grams)
To maintain weight	To maintain weight 3-4 servings (45-60 grams)
For active men	For active woman 4-5 servings (60-75 grams)

so will portion control help you lose weight. Try to use smaller plates and glasses—this is a natural way to control how much you eat.

Reduce calories. To lose weight, you need to burn more calories than you eat. Eating a more-nutritious diet will help you to reduce the number of calories you take in. Reduce your intake of fast food, soft drinks, and other processed and prepared foods—these foods are often high in calories and low in nutrients. Vegetables and whole grains are highly nutritious foods that tend to be lower in calories than many other choices.

Count carbs. The American Diabetes Association reports that more people lose weight when they follow a lower-carbohydrate diet. Determine how many carbohydrates you need daily based on how active you are.

Choose your drink carefully. Avoid sugared beverages. Also, note that energy drinks, sports drinks, and vitamin waters are frequently high in calories and low in nutrients. And, although 100 percent fruit juice is more nutritious than soda, it has approximately the same number of calories ounce for ounce. Try switching to water. It is calorie free and is the ultimate thirst-quencher. Or, as an alternate to drinking juice, eat whole, fresh fruit—in general, it has fewer calories than juice, and has plenty of healthful fiber.

Monitor progress. Chart your progress and stay accountable to your own goals by keeping daily track of the food and number of calories you eat, as well as your physical activity. Also keep track of your weight. Since your weight can fluctuate by a pound or two every day, it is more accurate to weigh yourself once a week, at the same time of day. This record can be a big help to motivate you with your weight-loss program. When you reach important goals, celebrate!

Get plenty of fiber. As mentioned earlier, fiber is an important part of a nutritious diet. But it can also help you lose weight. Although it has no calories, fiber helps you feel full because it adds bulk to your meal. If you are trying to lose weight, pay particular attention to selecting foods high in fiber. For example, even though real fruit juice has important nutrients, it's healthier to eat whole fruit instead, because fruit (including dried fruit) has fiber.

Overcoming Barriers to Success

Maintaining a positive attitude about your meal plan and weight control program is vital to your success. But, it is normal to "get off track" or feel discouraged once in a while. Here are some barriers you may encounter, along with tips to help you overcome them.

Trying to make major changes all at once. Realize you don't have to. Begin with focusing on eating regularly and balancing the amount of carbohydrates you eat throughout the day so that you maintain more-even levels of blood sugars. Fine tune your food plan as you learn more about balanced nutrition and blood sugar control.

Fearing change. Educate yourself. Learn about good nutrition and exercise. Once you fully understand which nutrients will help you be healthy and which foods are harmful, it will help motivate you to change your habits and stay on track.

Trying to do it alone. Seek support from your friends and family. Your doctor, health educator, and dietician should also be part of your support system. The good eating habits you will be adopting to help control your type 2 diabetes can also be beneficial for others in your household. If everyone in your home is eating more nutritiously, you can help each other stay on track.

Feeling all is lost if you get off track. Adopting nutritious eating habits is a process. Don't let a misstep get you off track. If you do find you've strayed from your meal plan, don't get bogged down in feeling all is hopeless. Focus on getting back onto your plan as soon as possible.

Being surrounded by food at work, at home, and at play. It's true—food is a big part of our world. We can sometimes feel surrounded by food, whether we are socializing or being influenced by advertisements we see on television. Although you can't do anything to change the number of food advertisements, you can do something about how you react to them. Start analyzing the food ads you see to notice what the advertiser is doing to pull you in. Having a critical eye when it comes to ads will help you stay on track.

Having a negative mind-set. To avoid the feeling that changing your lifestyle is a big pain, do things to make it fun:

- Make plans to cook nutritious meals with friends and family.
- Trade healthful recipes with friends and family.
- Be active doing something you enjoy, such as gardening, dancing, or taking walks with friends.

Changing Your Lifestyle

Adopting a healthier lifestyle means changing your habits in not only the way you eat, but in your attitude about food. Since you've acquired these habits over a lifetime, it will take some time to change them. But, by taking control of your lifestyle habits now, you will take control of your health and reduce your chances of developing the many complications that can result from type 2 diabetes.

Rule 3

Exercise Regularly

No doubt, you've heard about how important exercise is for everyone. If you've been diagnosed with type 2 diabetes, you've probably been told by your doctor that exercise is essential for managing the disease. But like many others, you may feel reluctant and unmotivated to start an ongoing exercise plan. All kinds of reasons may be popping into your head about why you can't exercise. You may tell yourself that you're too busy or that exercise has never seemed to help you in the past. Or maybe work and family obligations fill your week and you wonder where you'll find the time.

If you find yourself making excuses, it's time to reconsider the things you may be telling yourself about exercise. Many, many type 2 diabetes patients have felt just like you do about exercising. But by starting with a plan and starting slowly, they made progress. You can, too. And you'll soon find that, indeed, the benefits of exercise are many.

Benefits of Exercising

Improves Insulin Resistance

Physical exercise lowers blood sugars and improves insulin resistance. Very simply, exercise improves circulation and helps the body become more sensitive to insulin. This results in improved blood sugar levels. This benefit of increased sensitivity to insulin continues for hours after you stop exercising.

A sedentary lifestyle contributes to insulin resistance, and makes it more difficult to keep weight off. Even light or moderate physical activity can help lower blood sugars.

After you have been exercising for a while, when your weight comes down and your blood sugars improve, your doctor may even tell you that your diabetes medication dose can be reduced.

Promotes Weight Loss

Exercise burns calories. When you exercise regularly and maintain a balanced diet, your body will begin to burn more of the body's stored fat. Also, the more you exercise, the more your metabolism increases; this makes the body more efficient at burning excess fat. Exercise may also reduce appetite and food cravings.

Reduces Risk of Heart Disease and Lowers Blood Pressure

The heart is a muscle, and exercise makes it stronger. A stronger heart can pump more blood with less effort. Regular physical activity improves circulation, increases blood flow in the heart vessels, and improves the heart's overall efficiency. High blood pressure increases the risk of heart attack and stroke, but regular exercise will lower blood pressure.

Having a normal blood pressure also reduces the risk of kidney disease. High blood pressure can eventually damage blood vessels throughout the body, including those in the kidneys. If these blood vessels are damaged, they may no longer be effective in removing wastes and extra fluid from the body. Such extra fluid in the blood vessels may raise blood pressure even further.

Improves Cholesterol Levels

Improving cholesterol levels contributes to greater cardio-vascular health. Exercise does not burn off cholesterol like it does fat, but exercise can increase HDL cholesterol levels and reduce triglyceride and LDL cholesterol levels. Medical science is not entirely clear on how exercise improves cholesterol levels, but it's believed that aerobic exercise, such as walking, swimming, or biking, stimulates enzymes that affect the amount of cholesterol in the blood.

Studies suggest that regular exercise of at least thirty minutes a day and burning 800 to 1,200 calories a week may increase HDL cholesterol levels by as much as 3 to 5 percent. Similarly, this amount of exercise, along with a nutritious diet and weight control, has been shown to reduce triglycerides as much as 15 to 25 percent and reduce LDL cholesterol by as much as 5 to 10 percent.

Exercise may not produce improvements immediately. It may take several months for the improved cholesterol levels, also known as lipid levels, to show up in blood tests. Note that if you have a genetic trait that increases cholesterol levels, exercise may not be as effective in lowering cholesterol.

Increases Strength of Muscle and Bone

As we age, our muscle strength declines. After the age of thirty, we lose about five pounds of muscle each decade. If we don't engage in activities to strengthen and maintain muscles, we lose muscle mass and store more fat.

Exercise, both aerobic and strength training, increases muscle mass. Studies have proven that people who maintain their muscle mass have fewer disabilities when they become older.

Exercise also increases bone strength, as measured by bone mineral density, in people of all age groups. As we age, our bones become thinner and are more prone to breaking. Research shows that bone density can be increased with weight-bearing exercise. Talk to your doctor or diabetes educator for guidelines about how much weight you should be lifting and how frequently you should perform such exercise.

Strength training also stimulates the retention of calcium in the bones involved in the exercise. The degree to which bone strength improves depends on such factors as age, reproductive hormone status, nutrition, and the nature of the exercise.

Improves Flexibility

Exercise improves flexibility. Greater flexibility means greater range of motion; stronger muscles, bones, ligaments, and tendons; and better posture. All this helps our bodies move with greater ease and efficiency. Especially as we get older, our muscles become less pliable and some body movements become more difficult. For example, it may be more difficult to look over your shoulder or to bend over to tie your shoe. Greater flexibility reduces the risk of injuries such as those caused by falls.

Reduces Risk of Nerve Damage

High blood sugar levels can damage the body's intricate system of small blood vessels. Damage to these vessels can affect the eyes, the kidneys, and the body's extensive network of nerves, which involve functions such as heart rate, breathing, digestion, urination, glucose control, and perspiration. As explained earlier, exercise is one of the most effective ways to manage blood sugars.

Creates a Sense of Well-Being

Not only does exercise enhance physical health, but it also helps you feel better emotionally. When we exercise, the brain releases endorphins, hormones that are known to influence our moods. Exercise has been proven to decrease anxiety, anger, and depression, and even improve concentration and overall brain functioning. Exercise can also raise self-esteem by improving body image.

Reduces Tension and Stress

When we are stressed, our bodies become tight and tense and internally are preparing to take action. This is part of the body's natural flight or fight instinct. Part of this preparation involves the body making stored glucose available to cells for energy. As a result, more glucose enters the bloodstream. Exercise reduces stress, and in turn, improves insulin's efficiency and relaxes muscles.

Starting an Exercise Program

Starting an exercise program is probably not as difficult as you think it might be. The most difficult part is putting the plan into action. Pace yourself. You may want to do too much too soon. If so, you may need to adjust the way you think about exercising. You don't have to be running a five-mile race to be exercising. Nor is it required that you visit a gym several times a week. Instead, you can develop a personal activity plan that fits your lifestyle.

Here's another key point to remember: Once you start exercising regularly, within a very short period of time you will feel the benefits. Most people are amazed at how much better they feel.

Once you've made the decision to start an exercise program, it helps to set goals.

Set Goals for Success

Research clearly points out that your chances of continuing and succeeding with an exercise regimen increase significantly if you set goals. Many diabetes educators use the S.M.A.R.T guidelines for setting exercise and weight-loss goals. The guidelines are as follows:

- **S:** *Specific.* Keep goals specific. For example, you may want to set a goal to lose ten pounds rather than say, "I want to lose weight."
- **M:** *Measurable.* Keep goals measurable. Keep track of your exercise sessions so you can measure your progress.
- **A:** *Attainable.* Set goals that are attainable. Keep them simple and practical.
- **R:** *Realistic.* Keep goals realistic. Don't try to make up for years of inactivity in a short amount of time.
- **T:** *Timely.* Set a time or date for reaching the goal. Without a goal date, your chances for success decrease.

Set both short-term and long-term goals. Almost any goal can be reached if broken into small steps. For example, you might start with a goal to lose five pounds rather than fifty pounds.

Start small and build from there. Take notice of even the smallest amount of progress you are making, and be patient and encouraging with yourself.

Writing down your goals helps keep you accountable to yourself and helps you stay motivated. Write your goal on a note card and stick it on your refrigerator!

Your Exercise Program

What kind of exercise should you do? There is no one-size-fits-all answer. Do things you enjoy. Explore the possibilities. Do a variety of things—you don't need to stick with only one type of exercise. You can ask your healthcare provider, a diabetes educator, or a personal trainer to help you get started with an exercise program that is right for you. These professionals will explain the types of exercises that are appropriate for you; they will also give you their recommendations on intensity levels, duration, and frequency of exercise.

A good, all-around exercise plan will include aerobic exercise, strength training, and flexibility exercises. Gaining a better understanding of these exercises will help you set up a good plan of action.

Aerobic Exercise

Sometimes referred to as endurance training or cardiovascular exercise, aerobic exercise is physical activity that increases the need for oxygen. It increases your heart rate and makes your heart work more efficiently. Aerobic exercise has proven to be the most beneficial type of activity for preventing heart disease. Exercise that falls into this category includes activities such as walking, dancing, jogging, hiking, cycling, and swimming. Here are tips for aerobic exercising:

- Don't wait until you *feel* like starting. Set a routine and start to follow it.
- If you find an activity you enjoy, you'll be more likely to continue it.
- Start slowly. Begin with five to ten minutes a day, several days a week.
- Gradually increase your exercising to thirty minutes a day, five days a week.
- As you exercise, take the "talk test." If you can't talk without gasping, slow down.
- If you miss a day, don't think you've failed. Just start again tomorrow.

Strength Training

Strength training, also called resistance training, is the use of resistance against muscles to build up muscle strength. There are many different methods of strength training, but common ones include weight lifting or stretching elastic bands. The following are tips for strength training:

- Stretch your muscles before strength-training exercises.
- Start slowly. Build up to fifteen- to thirty-minute sessions twice a week.
- Talk to a health professional or trainer about the amount of weight you should lift.
- First work on large muscles—thighs, back, chest. These take more energy.
- Work last on smaller muscles—triceps, biceps, forearms. They require less energy.
- Allow at least forty-eight hours of rest between strength-training sessions. On days you're not doing strength training, do aerobic workouts.

Flexibility Exercises

Flexibility exercises involve slow, controlled stretching of the muscles. Stretching should become an important part of every exercise session. Here are tips for flexibility exercises:

- Perform stretching of major muscle groups two to three times a week, and keep your routine consistent.
- When you stretch, breathe deeply and fully.
- Stretch in a slow, controlled manner.
- Hold stretches for ten to thirty seconds. Do not bounce—it can cause injury.
- Pay attention to your body. Don't overdo it. If you feel pain, slow down and move more easily into the stretch. Stop if pain persists.
- Don't overlook the importance of stretching as a form of exercise.

How Much Exercise Do You Need?

Some experts recommend walking for thirty minutes daily. Others suggest walking for twenty minutes three times a week. Yet others suggest getting a pedometer, which measures the number of steps you take, and keep track of how many steps you take each day. How many steps should you aim for daily? The average person's stride length is approximately 2.5 feet long. That means it takes just over 2,000 steps to walk one mile. Any of these approaches will benefit you.

Surgeon General's Recommendations

The Surgeon General's Report on Physical Activity and Health recommends that most adults should accumulate thirty minutes of moderate-intensity activities on most days of the week. Here, the word "accumulate" means you need not do the exercise all at one time. Rather, you might divide the time into ten- to fifteen-minute periods during the day. The report defines "moderate intensity" as feeling warm and slightly out of breath as you perform the exercise.

ADA Recommendations

The American Diabetes Association recommends that people with diabetes aim for 150 minutes of exercise each week at moderate intensity, such as walking. You can divide up those minutes any way you wish; for example, you may wish to exercise 30 minutes a day five days a week or 50 minutes a day three days a week.

In addition to walking, you may want to include any number of other activities, including gardening, doing yard work, swimming, or bicycling. The list is virtually limitless. The goal is to engage in any activity that increases your heart rate and causes you to break a light sweat.

Any of your daily living activities could count as physical activity. For example, instead of circling the parking lot for ten minutes searching for the parking spot closest to the store door, park as far away from the store as possible and walk. Another simple idea: commit to taking the stairs instead of the elevator or escalator whenever possible. Chores around the home count, too. If you are mowing the lawn or vacuuming the house, you can include these activities in your activity minutes for the day.

Check Blood Sugar Levels before Exercise

It's important to check your blood sugar levels before you exercise. Exercise of moderate intensity may cause your blood sugars to drop by as much as 50 points for every thirty minutes you exercise. If you check your blood sugars before exercising and you're at 150 mg/dl, your blood sugar level may drop to about 100 mg/dl. If your blood sugar level is already 100 mg/dl before you exercise, it may drop too low after you begin exercising. In this case, before you exercise, you'll want to eat a one-carbohydrate snack—a piece of bread, a piece of fruit, or a granola bar.

Most people whose blood sugars are running higher are pleased to see their blood sugars drop after exercise; however, it's important to know that vigorous exercise can also cause blood sugars to rise temporarily. If this occurs, test again thirty minutes later.

If you're exercising for a long period of time, it's a good idea to check your blood sugar levels before, during, and after your workout to make sure you avoid any dangerous swings in levels. This is especially true if you take insulin. If your blood sugars drop to 70 mg/dl or below during exercise, ingest a source of quick carbohydrates such as fruit juice or regular soda. Many people with diabetes carry glucose tablets with them and take two to five tablets when they need a source of quick glucose.

When Not to Exercise

Delay exercise if your glucose level is at 300 mg/dl or more since vigorous exercise can temporarily make blood sugars go higher. Why is this important? If your pre-exercise glucose is more than 250 mg/dl, you could experience the acute symptoms of high blood sugar levels, including excessive thirst, which leads to increased water intake and excessive urination. This can lead to dehydration if blood sugar levels are not decreased. As a general rule, bring your blood sugar levels down before exercising.

Other Safety Precautions

Before you set your new exercise program in motion, you will need to take some precautionary measures. First, talk to your doctor or diabetes educator about the type of exercise plan that is appropriate for you. It's important to determine whether it's safe for you to exercise vigorously. If you have cardiovascular risks, are over the age of thirty-five, or if you have been sedentary up until now, you should receive a thorough medical evaluation.

Your doctor will likely review your medical history and perform a physical examination, which may include a stress test. For a stress test, electrodes are attached to your chest and you walk on a treadmill so your doctor can see how your heart responds to exertion. Your doctor may also want an *echocardiogram* of your heart; this is a noninvasive diagnostic procedure that uses ultrasound to study the structure and motions of the heart. These tests tell the doctor whether your heart is receiving adequate blood flow during exercise. If you are not able to walk on a treadmill, your doctor may substitute a medication to increase your heart rate. (If your walking is impaired, your doctor may also have suggestions for other types of exercise.)

When you exercise, especially if you're not close to home, it's a good idea to carry a medical ID, indicating that you have type 2 diabetes, in case you experience any medical problems. Take along some high-carbohydrate snacks or glucose tablets in case your blood sugar level drops and you begin to feel weak. Consider working out with a friend, who'll be with you if you need help of any kind.

Your clothing should be comfortable and appropriate for the type of activity you have chosen. Wear comfortable, supportive shoes and clean, dry socks; if you've had any complications, such as sores on your feet, check with your doctor about your exercise plan. If you are planning to exercise outside, avoid temperatures that are extremely hot or cold. Also, make sure you drink plenty of water before, during, and after your workout.

Include Warm-Ups and Cool-Downs

Always do at least a five-minute warm-up before exercising and do a five-minute cool-down afterward. Warm-ups should include an exercise that slightly raises your heart rate and blood pressure so that you're preparing your body for the activity you are about to perform. Usually, the warm-up would be a lighter, slower version of the activity you will be doing, such as walking. For the warm-up, you'd walk at a slower pace. The cool-down is based on the same concept; after walking vigorously, walk slowly to cool down. The intention is to avoid any drastic changes in heart rate and blood pressure in a short amount of time; this is better for your heart and will prevent dizziness.

Commit to Exercise

Exercise is not something that just happens to us. We need to make it happen. If you're going to integrate exercise into your life, you need to schedule it. Commit to it and carve out the time for it. Just as brushing your teeth and taking a shower are daily rituals, exercise can become a familiar ritual.

Regardless of whatever excuses for not exercising run through your mind, it's time to reframe how you think about exercise. Exercise is not the enemy. If you have type 2 diabetes, exercise can become your best friend—one that can dramatically improve your health.

Rule 4

Monitor Blood
Sugar Levels

If you have type 2 diabetes, it's important to test your glucose levels regularly. In fact, testing is essential for controlling your diabetes. Each time you test, you obtain a snapshot of your blood glucose level. Regular testing will help you understand factors that influence your blood sugar levels and having this knowledge will help you determine what to do when your blood sugar levels are too high or too low. People with diabetes who regularly monitor their blood sugar tend to enjoy better overall health and avoid complications.

To test your blood sugar level, you'll use a small device called a *glucometer* or glucose meter. This test involves using a small needle, called a lancet, to draw a drop of blood, usually by pricking your finger with the lancet. Then, you apply the drop of blood to a test strip. Within a few seconds, the glucometer gives you a reading of your current glucose level.

Choosing a Glucose Meter

When you shop for a glucose meter, you'll find nearly two dozen models on the market. They offer various features, ranging from those that allow you to draw blood from places other than your fingers to those that "speak," giving you audio test results. Some meters allow you to store additional data such as exercise, health, food, and medical information. Your doctor, diabetes educator, or pharmacist can help you understand the various meters and the options they offer.

Your insurance provider may require that you buy a certain model of glucose meter if it is to cover the expense. You also may want to check with local diabetes education centers; they often provide free meters and, in return, you buy testing strips for the brand of meter you receive. Finally, you may save money by ordering your meter and testing supplies from companies online.

Using Your Glucose Meter

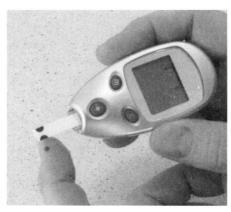

Initially, the idea of drawing blood may seem unpleasant. You may feel overwhelmed, upset, and even angry. And you may be apprehensive or fearful about drawing blood from your finger or other site on your body. You're not alone. These feelings are normal—many people feel this way at first. However, most people with diabetes quickly learn to master the task of testing their glucose and do not find it painful.

When checking glucose levels, prick the side of your finger to avoid the sensitive nerves in the fingertips.

Before you begin using your glucose meter, read the manufacturer's instructions. Determine whether you need to test on your finger or if you can test on an alternate site such as the forearm, hand, or thigh. If you do test on your finger, note that the tips of the fingers are filled with nerve endings and pricking the skin in this area with a needle may be slightly painful. Instead, prick the side of your fingertip where there are fewer nerve endings.

Here are guidelines for using your glucose meter:

- If you are testing on your finger or hand, wash your hands with soap and warm water. Hold your hand down below your waist for a few seconds to increase blood flow to the fingers. If you are testing another site, clean the area with an alcohol swab.
- Insert an unused test strip into the glucose meter.
- Insert a clean lancet into the lancing device. The lancing device is spring-loaded. The spring forces the lancet to prick the skin to obtain a drop of blood.
- Lance your finger and, if necessary, gently squeeze until a drop of blood forms.
- Touch the edge of the test strip to the blood and wait for the result.
- The blood glucose level will appear in the meter's display window.

If Readings Appear Inaccurate

Several factors can affect the accuracy of the readings you get from your glucose meter. If you suspect your reading is inaccurate, review the following steps:

- *Glucose meter.* Make sure the meter is at room temperature. Verify that the test window and strip guide are clean and free of blood. Replace the meter batteries if necessary.
- *Test strips.* Discard outdated or damaged strips. Always store the strips according to the manufacturer's instructions. For example, keep strips away from heat, light, and air when not in use. Exposure to air will decrease the enzyme activity in the test strips, making them ineffective for testing.
- *Coding.* Some glucometers require the user to manually enter a code found on the vial of test strips. If your meter must be coded to the test strips, check the code number on the test strips container and make

Goals for Blood Sugar Levels

Testing time	Target range
Fasting	90-130 mg/dl
Before a meal	70-130 mg/dl
After a meal (two hours)	less than 180 mg/dl
At bedtime	110-140 mg/dl

sure your meter is set to the code. By entering the coding or chip into the glucose meter, the meter will be calibrated to that batch of test strips. Having a wrong code can give you inaccurate readings.

- *Testing site.* If you use alcohol to clean your skin at the test site, be sure to wipe away the first drop of blood before collecting the subsequent drop for testing.
- *Retesting.* To retest, apply a drop of blood to the test strip and test again. You may also want to try using a new test strip.

If you experience problems with your meter, check the manual that came with the device for information. Also, you may find a toll-free number on the back of the meter so you can call the manufacturer to ask for help.

A word about disposal of used needles: Always dispose of these items carefully to avoid the risk of anyone accidentally pricking a finger. Many pharmacies have a "sharps" dispenser for customers to discard used needles. In some communities, supervised disposal service is available.

How Often Should You Test?

The amount of glucose in the blood varies from hour to hour. Daily monitoring is the best way to keep track of how food, physical activity, and other factors affect your blood sugars. Shortly after you are diagnosed with type 2 diabetes, your doctor or diabetes educator will likely advise you to check your blood sugars several times throughout the day. The most common patterns for blood sugar monitoring include testing:

- when fasting, usually upon rising in the morning
- before meals
- two hours after meals
- at bedtime

Once you begin to understand your blood sugar patterns, you can rotate the timing of blood sugar testing each day. This will allow you to perform fewer tests. For example, by rotating your testing schedule, you might check your blood sugars before breakfast and before your evening meal on one day; then check it before lunch and at bedtime the next day. With this schedule, you will be checking only two times per day, but you are monitoring results over four time periods. You can ask your healthcare provider for guidance on how often to check your blood sugars.

Understanding Your Glucose Test Results

The blood sugar values listed in the "Goals for Blood Sugar Levels" table are recommendations and should not be inter-preted as strict guidelines for everyone. Your physician will help you establish your own personal target range for blood sugar levels.

The fasting blood sugar level, taken when you get up in the morning, tells you about your blood sugar levels during the night. The blood sugar reading before a meal is typically most relevant to individuals who are using insulin. Some patients adjust their insulin dosages depending on premeal readings.

Your sugar level two hours after a meal, also referred to as a two-hour *postprandial* blood sugar level, tells you how the foods you ate affected your glucose. If the blood sugar value is high, you most likely ate too much or you ate the wrong foods; it could also indicate that you require more medication to control blood sugars.

Blood Glucose Log	Breakfast		Lunch		Dinner		Bedtime	
	Fasting	2 Hours After	Before	2 Hours After	Before	2 Hours After	Before	2 Hours After
Monday								
Tuesday								
Wednesday								
Thursday								
Friday								
Saturday								
Sunday								

Bedtime testing gives you a reading of blood sugars several hours after your evening meal. If blood sugars are high, it is a good idea to review the amount of food you ate as well as whether you are taking the correct dose of medication. If your blood sugars are low, it will help you determine whether your insulin or oral medication dose is appropriate or whether you should eat a snack to restore your blood sugar levels.

Emotional Reactions

It's normal for blood glucose readings to trigger strong feelings. You may feel positive and upbeat when blood glucose values fall into the target range, but get frustrated when the values are high. Remember that the target range is a tool to help you assess the effectiveness of your daily diabetes treatment plan. It provides valuable information for adjusting your plan as necessary. The goal of glucose management is not to be perfect, but rather to remain within the target range as often as possible to maintain your health and prevent future complications.

Keeping a Food Diary

It will help if you keep a food diary of what you eat each day, especially when you first start testing your sugar levels. This will help you learn which foods cause the most fluctuations in your blood sugars. In time, you'll develop a better overall picture of which foods are best for you and which foods to avoid.

Recording Test Results

In addition to keeping a food diary, you'll benefit from keeping a log of your blood sugar test results. This will be valuable in helping you identify patterns in the rise and fall of your blood sugars. For example, you will learn how skipping meals, eating high-carbohydrate meals, and exercising or not exercising affects your blood sugars.

You may have received a log book for keeping track of your daily blood sugar levels when you purchased your glucose meter. Or you may want to develop a logbook similar to the one shown on page 58.

Hemoglobin A1c Blood Tests

In addition to monitoring your blood sugar levels daily, you and your doctor will periodically test your hemoglobin A1c levels. As mentioned earlier, this test is not influenced by daily fluctuations in your blood glucose concentration; instead it provides your average glucose levels over the last three months.

The lower the A1c value, the better the blood sugar control. An A1c value of 6 percent indicates an average daily blood sugar level of roughly 115 mg/dl. An A1c value of 9 percent indicates a higher average blood sugar level of 210 mg/dl. Your doctor will determine the A1c level that provides you the greatest health benefit.

Hemoglobin A1c: What the Numbers Mean	
If Your A1c Is:	Your Average Blood Sugar Is:
4	50
5	80
6	115
7	150
8	180
9	210
10	245
11	280
12	310
13	345

A1c testing kits also are available for home use without a prescription; however, home test kits may not be as accurate as tests performed in clinical laboratories.

Factors Affecting Blood Sugar Levels

Numerous factors affect how the body metabolizes glucose. The following are factors most likely to cause blood sugars to rise, fall, or remain steady throughout the day.

Diet. As stressed earlier, diet plays a crucial role in the management of your blood sugars. Don't skip meals. Strive to be consistent with your food intake—eat similar amounts of food at the same times each day. Also, try to eat the same recommended amount of carbohydrates at each meal to avoid swings in blood sugars throughout the day. Carbohydrates have a greater impact on your blood sugars than protein or fat.

Exercise. If you test your blood sugar level before and after exercise, you'll readily see how exercise can lower blood sugars. Four to six hours after exercise, your muscles continue to recover and absorb glucose, resulting in lowered levels. Your blood sugar levels may be affected if you have not eaten enough carbohydrates or if you're not taking the correct dosage of diabetes medications that has been matched to your food intake and the amount of exercise you do.

Stress. Stress affects blood sugar levels. Two scenarios are most common. First, when under stress, you may abandon your regular routine, not eat well, exercise infrequently, and skip blood sugar checks. Second, when you are stressed, your body may produce hormones that prevent insulin from working properly, thereby causing blood sugar levels to rise. If you note a correlation between stress and higher blood sugar levels, discuss this with your doctor or diabetes educator.

Illness and injury. Illness and injury can present special challenges if you have diabetes. When you're sick or injured, your body produces hormones to fight the illness. These hormones may cause blood sugar levels to rise. Continue to monitor your blood sugars frequently. Try to stick to your regular eating plan. If you are eating less than usual, your doctor may instruct you to temporarily adjust your diabetes medication to avoid dangerously low blood sugars. If you suffer from nausea or vomiting, contact your doctor.

Alcoholic beverages. Drinking alcohol may cause your blood sugar levels to fall too low. Even as little as two ounces can cause this effect. If you choose to drink, do so in moderation. Never drink on an empty stomach or when your blood sugar level is already low. And, only drink alcohol with food. Keep in mind that drinking alcohol also may cause your blood sugar levels to rise, especially if sugary sodas and fruit juices are

The "15-15 Rule" for Treating Low Blood Sugars

If your blood sugars drop below 70 mg/dl, take these steps:

- Consume 15 grams of carbohydrates.
- Wait 15 minutes, then check your blood sugars again.
- If your blood sugars are still below 70 mg/dl, eat 15 more grams of carbohydrates.
- Wait another 15 minutes and check your blood sugars again.
- Repeat these steps until your blood sugar level is above 70 mg/dl.
- If your blood sugars don't rise and you have a problem staying alert, call 911 or have someone call for you.

mixed with the alcohol. Light beer and dry wines contain fewer calories and carbohydrates than other alcoholic drinks. Always monitor your blood sugars before and after you drink alcohol.

Prescription medications. Taking your diabetes medication at the same time each day and keeping food intake consistent each day will help you keep blood sugar levels consistent. If you take your diabetes medication and consume too little food, you may experience low blood sugars, or *hypoglycemia.* The reverse also holds: Eat too much food, and you may experience a rise in blood sugars, or *hyperglycemia.*

Also, be aware of the impact of other prescription drugs on your body. When your doctor prescribes a new medication for a condition other than diabetes, ask how the new medication may affect your blood sugar levels. For example, both steroids (used for arthritis and other diseases) and beta blockers (used for some heart conditions) are known to raise blood sugars. If the new medications cause your blood sugar levels to rise, tell your doctor.

Hormone levels. The following factors may cause hormone levels to fluctuate and blood sugar levels to rise: menstruation, birth control pills, menopause, and hormone replacement therapy in menopausal women.

Managing Hypoglycemia

We've discussed factors that influence your blood sugars daily. If your blood sugar levels fall too low, you develop a condition called hypoglycemia. It may bring on any of the following symptoms:

- weakness
- shakiness
- irritability
- dizziness

- hunger
- headache
- confusion
- cold sweat

If you feel like you have hypoglycemia, check your blood sugar level. If your level is below 70 mg/dl, follow the "15-15 Rule," which explains how to raise your blood sugars.

You can get 15 grams of carbohydrates from a number of sources, including one-half cup of fruit juice, a cup of nonfat or low-fat milk, or two to four glucose tablets.

Note that there is a lag between the time you eat the carbo-hydrates and the time your blood sugar level rises. Don't panic. It's far better to eat a few carbohydrates every fifteen minutes and wait for results than to consume too many carbohydrates quickly and experience high blood sugars for an extended period of time.

Managing Hyperglycemia

The same factors that may cause glucose levels to fall can often cause glucose levels to *rise*. If your blood sugar levels are too high, you are said to have hyperglycemia. Symptoms of hyperglycemia include:

- increased thirst or hunger
- frequent urination
- tingling in hands or feet
- slow-healing sores

- feeling tired
- stomach pain or nausea
- dry or itchy skin
- frequent infections

The best way to avoid hyperglycemia is to follow your diet and exercise plan and visit your doctor regularly.

The Dawn Effect

Some people experience what's called the "dawn effect," which refers to an exaggerated increase in blood sugars that occurs between the hours of 2 A.M. and 8 A.M. The dawn effect is caused by the body's early-morning spike in growth hormones and cortisol, which affect blood sugars. Your doctor may advise you to avoid late-night eating or he or she may adjust your medication.

When to Contact Your Doctor

If your blood sugar level is frequently too low or too high, talk to your doctor about modifying your diabetes medication, meal plan, or activity level. Finally, contact your doctor if you encounter any of the following situations:

- Your blood sugar level is persistently above the target range you and your doctor have established.
- Your blood sugar level is higher than normal during an illness. The degree of glucose elevation may indicate the severity of illness or infection.
- You have a blood sugar reaction and require help from another person.
- Your blood sugar levels are frequently too low (hypoglycemia).

Commit to Routine Blood Sugar Checks

Managing type 2 diabetes is a daily commitment. Routine blood glucose monitoring will serve you as a very important guide—one that helps you determine the actions you need to take to control of your blood sugar levels.

Rule 5

Take Medications as Directed

Most individuals diagnosed with type 2 diabetes take medications as one of the methods for controlling their blood sugar levels. Together with proper diet and exercise, these drugs are vital to their long-term health and well-being.

Drug therapies for type 2 diabetes come in pill form or in the form of injections that you give yourself. The wide variety of medications now available means that your doctor can prescribe medications or combinations of medications that are tailored to your individual needs.

Oral Medications

Your doctor will prescribe medication based on your blood glucose levels. Whether they are pills or injectable drugs, all of the type 2 diabetes medications used to control blood sugars will do one or more of the following:

- Help your body produce more of its own insulin
- Reduce the amount of sugar produced by your own body
- Reduce the rate at which blood sugars can rise in your bloodstream
- Help your body use insulin more efficiently

Usually, oral medications are considered the first line of defense against unstable blood sugar levels. However, depending on your circumstance, a combination of oral medications and insulin may be the best option. In fact, it is becoming more and more common for people with type 2 diabetes to be on a combination of medications. Over time, the course of treatment may also mean being prescribed different medications as well as different doses.

Oral medications for type 2 diabetes are grouped into six different "classes," based on their chemical makeup and how they work. The six classes, listed in the order in which they are most commonly prescribed, include:

- biguanides
- sulfonylureas
- thiazolidinediones (TZDs)
- DPP-4 inhibitors
- meglitinides
- alpha-glucosidase inhibitors

Biguanides

Biguanides are among the most commonly prescribed medications for people who have just been diagnosed with type 2 diabetes. Biguanides reduce the amount of sugar produced by your liver. In addition, they make your body more sensitive to insulin so that your body's cells absorb glucose more readily. Together, these effects cause reductions in blood glucose levels.

It is likely you will start with a medication called *metformin*. It has few side effects and is available in generic forms, so it is less expensive than some similar drugs.

Possible side effects are: diarrhea, nausea, and vomiting. These side effects are usually short-lived. Metformin is not recommended for patients with liver, kidney, or heart failure. Commonly prescribed biguanides include: metformin (*Glucophage, Riomet, Fortamet, Glumetza*).

Sulfonylureas

Sulfonylureas stimulate cells in your pancreas, where insulin is produced, to increase the production of insulin. The more insulin you have in your body, the more glucose is moved into cells and absorbed, lowering blood sugar levels. A variety of sulfonylureas are available; their differences are related to the frequency with which you take them, interactions with other medications, and their side effects.

Possible side effects are: hypoglycemia, nausea, upset stomach or heartburn, skin rash or itching, and weight gain. Commonly prescribed sulfonylureas include: glyburide (*Diabeta, Micronase, Glynase, PresTab*); glipizide (*Glucotrol, Glucotrol XL*); and glimepiride (*Amaryl*).

Thiazolidinediones (TZDs)

TZDs lower blood glucose levels primarily by improving the effectiveness of the body's tissues using the insulin already on hand. This means that the insulin your body makes is more efficient at lowering glucose levels.

Possible side effects are: weight gain, fluid retention, and osteoporosis (loss of bone density, which results in more fragile bones). TZDs are not recommended for patients with congestive heart failure. Commonly prescribed TZDs include: pioglitazone (*Actos*) and rosiglitazone (*Avandia*).

Although TZDs are effective at controlling blood glucose, one of them, *Avandia*, has been associated with heart attack and other potentially fatal cardiovascular events. Although these problems have been recognized by the Food and Drug Administration (FDA) as persistent, the FDA has not found them to be pervasive enough to take *Avandia* off the market.

DPP-4 Inhibitors

Through a complex series of actions, DPP-4 inhibitors work through multiple mechanisms to improve blood glucose levels. It is known that hormones produced from the stomach when we're eating actually work to increase insulin secretion. One of these hormones, called glucagon-like peptide-1 (GLP-1), increases insulin in response to rising glucose and also slows down the rate of carbohydrate absorption at meals.

An enzyme, Dipeptidyl peptidase-4 (DPP-4), breaks down GLP-1. This class of medications inhibits DPP-4 in order to increase the amount of naturally occurring GLP-1 in your body. These agents are a newer class of oral drugs that may be used individually or in combination with other pills.

Possible side effects are: common cold, upper respiratory infection, stomach pain, and diarrhea. Commonly prescribed DPP-4 inhibitors include: sitagliptin (*Januvia*) and saxagliptin (*Onglyza*).

Meglitinides

Like sulfonylureas, meglitinides also increase the secretion of insulin by the pancreas. However, with meglitinides, this effect is rapid and short-lived. These drugs are taken with meals so that the short burst of insulin can immediately stimulate your cells to absorb glucose at the time when your blood sugar levels are highest—right after you've eaten. The primary shortcoming of these drugs is that they are inefficient compared to other, more potent glucose-lowering drugs. However, if you are very active and your blood sugar levels are not too high, these drugs might be right for you.

Possible side effects are: mild hypoglycemia, upper respiratory tract infection, and weight gain. Commonly prescribed meglitinides include: repaglinide (*Prandin*) and nateglinide (*Starlix*).

Alpha-Glucosidase Inhibitors

These medications slow the process of digestion, and therefore slow down the rate at which glucose enters the bloodstream. These medications are taken at mealtimes. They are almost always taken in combination with other diabetes medications. The biggest problem with these drugs is that they have a potent effect on the gastrointestinal system. Due to the way they slow digestion, these medications result in additional sugar in the colon. When normal intestinal bacteria digest these sugars, gas is produced. This side effect is frequently unacceptable to individuals who try these medications.

Possible side effects are: diarrhea and gas. Commonly prescribed alpha-glucosidase inhibitors include: acarbose (*Precose*) and miglitol (*Glyset*).

Combination Medications

As time goes by, some people with type 2 diabetes need more than one type of medication. In deciding whether you'll need additional medication, your doctor will first consider how well the medications you are currently taking are working. If your blood sugars are not under control, you will likely need a second medication.

Some of the oral medications available come in combination form so that you get two medications in one pill. One of the advantages of combination pills is that you have fewer pills to take. However, combination pills often cost more than other medications.

Non-Insulin Injections

Many people who do not yet need insulin benefit from non-insulin medications that are injected. There are two such drugs that help reduce blood sugar levels. These drugs are considered "add-ons" to oral medications. If you are not meeting your blood glucose goals with your existing oral medications, these injectable drugs may be helpful.

Incretin Mimetics

Taken at mealtimes, *incretin mimetics* slow the process of digestion, and therefore slow the rate at which glucose from digested foods enters the bloodstream. This drug has a potent ability to increase insulin. It also acts as an appetite suppressant and can contribute to weight loss. Although some of the side effects can be unpleasant, many people find them to be temporary.

Possible side effects are: hypoglycemia, nausea, diarrhea, and weight loss. Commonly prescribed incretin mimetics include: exenatide (*Byetta*) and liraglutide (*Victoza*).

Synthetic Amylin Hormone

One of the primary actions of this medication is to improve the effectiveness of your body's own insulin. However, this drug's ability to lower glucose may not be as great as that of other medications. In addition, because it is an appetite suppressant, synthetic amylin hormone is associated with weight loss.

Possible side effects are: nausea, weight loss, and hypoglycemia. A commonly prescribed synthetic amylin hormone is pramlintide (*Symlin*).

When Do You Need Insulin Therapy?

You probably wonder if or when you will need insulin therapy. Over the course of years, the majority of people with type 2 diabetes will eventually need insulin injections. There is no specific timeline to follow. It's time to start injections when oral medications are no longer effective in maintaining tight blood sugar controls.

Initially, you may be anxious or fearful about giving yourself injections. This is a normal reaction—most people feel the same way. However, your doctor, nurse, or diabetes educator will instruct you as to how to give yourself the injections. Most type 2 diabetes patients quickly learn how to inject themselves, and most report that the injections are not painful.

Insulin Injections

Insulin is the most potent drug available for lowering glucose levels. However, if it were used in pill form, it would be destroyed during the digestion process. As a result, insulin must be taken by injection. Insulin comes in several forms, which are classified based on how quickly the insulin starts to work and how long its effects last.

Insulin's *onset* refers to the length of time it takes for insulin to reach the bloodstream and begin lowering blood sugars. The *peak time* refers to the period of time in which the insulin is doing the maximum amount of work to lower blood sugars. The length of time the insulin continues to lower blood sugars is called the *duration*.

Long-Acting and Rapid-Acting Insulin

To better understand the type of insulin injections you may need, it will help to understand the two ways in which the body uses insulin. First, the body uses insulin slowly to deliver glucose to cells around the clock in order to maintain cellular functioning. This is called *basal* insulin, or "long-acting insulin." Second, the body also uses insulin in quick, short bursts, delivering glucose to the body's cells when glucose has been released into the bloodstream in high levels. This would be the case after a meal. This type of insulin is referred to as *bolus*, or "rapid-acting" insulin.

The insulin your doctor prescribes may be long-acting or rapid-acting. Long-acting insulin provides a continuous level of insulin, much like a normal pancreas would. Rapid-acting insulin is effective in controlling blood sugars after a meal. Most doctors prefer to adjust the doses of these two types of insulin separately; however, a prescribed, premixed combination of the two types of insulin is available. Individuals who have problems with vision or have difficulty giving themselves injections may benefit from the premixed insulin.

Once you begin your insulin therapy, you will be asked to monitor your blood sugar levels regularly and report them to your healthcare provider so that dosage adjustments can be made if necessary. As a general rule, your doctor will have you start with a prescription for a lower level of insulin in order to avoid hypoglycemia. Your prescription dose will likely be increased eventually, based on your blood sugar levels.

Possible side effects of insulin are: hypoglycemia and allergic reaction (rash or itching) at the injection site. Commonly prescribed long-acting insulins include: glargine (*Lantus*); detemir (*Levemir*); and NPH (*Humulin N, Novolin N*).

Commonly prescribed rapid-acting insulins include: lispro (*Humolog*); aspart (*NovoLog*); glulisine (*Apidra*); and regular human insulin (*Humulin R, Novolin R*).

71

Insulin Delivery Methods

Your healthcare professional will instruct you on how to give yourself insulin injections. The three available methods are needle injection, insulin pens, and insulin pumps.

Needle injection. Insulin is given by injection with a syringe and needle that is directed into the fleshy soft tissue. Syringes come in sizes of 30, 50, and 100 units. The needles are extremely fine, which reduces any sensation of pain.

Insulin pens. An insulin pen, about the size of a ballpoint pen, comes with a prefilled insulin cartridge. Prior to injection, you insert a short, fine, disposable needle into the tip of the pen. The pen has a dial for selecting the correct dosage. You press a button at the end of the pen to deliver the injection just under the skin.

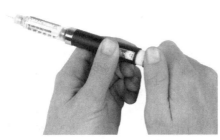

Insulin pens are convenient and easy to use. The pen may be a good choice for children who are old enough to administer their own insulin. It's also convenient for people who are busy and on the go, as well as for those who have visual or motor impairments. Although insulin pens are growing in popularity in the United States, they are more commonly used in other countries.

An insulin injection pen resembles a large pen. It uses cartridges of insulin and disposable needles

Insulin pumps. An insulin pump is a small device that dispenses insulin through a small catheter. The pump itself, about the size of a deck of cards, may be attached to a belt or pocket. A pump eliminates the need for repeated injections, and it allows for flexibility in eating times. When you're ready to eat, you press a button and the pump releases a preset dose of insulin.

The location of the catheter should be moved to a different site every few days. Your physician will teach you how to insert the catheter. Insulin pumps are more expensive than standard needles and syringes, and are not always covered by insurance plans.

Your Insulin Routine

No matter the type of insulin therapy you're prescribed, it's important to establish a routine. Your insulin routine will include where you inject, called the injection site; the timing of injections; and the storage of your insulin.

Injection sites. The insulin should be injected into the fat layer just under the skin. If it is injected into muscle, the insulin is absorbed too fast. You may inject insulin in the abdomen, backs of the upper arms, buttocks, hip areas, and in the front and sides of the thighs.

Compared to other sites, injecting in the abdomen is the preferred injection site because the insulin enters the blood-

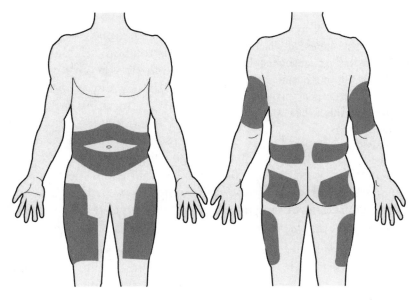

Insulin injections may be given in the shaded areas shown above—abdomen, backs of the upper arms, buttocks, hip areas, and in the front and sides of the thighs.

73

stream faster, the abdomen provides a larger surface for rotating the injection points, and changes in blood flow to the abdomen after exercise are less dramatic than at other injections sites. (Blood flow affects absorption rates.)

Avoid injecting yourself in the exact same spot, which is called the "injection point," each time you give yourself an injection. (Note: Injection *site* refers to the area of the body in which injections may be given. The injection *point* refers to the exact place on the skin where you insert the needle.) Repeated injections at the same injection point can result in a condition called *lipohypertrophy*, which is the buildup of fatty tissue. In addition to creating unsightly lumps, this condition can slow the rate at which insulin enters the bloodstream.

> ### Coordinate Meals and Medication
>
> Coordinate your meals and your diabetes medication. If you haven't eaten when you take your medication, insulin medications especially, your blood sugars may drop to levels that are dangerously low. If you have eaten too much prior to taking your medications, your blood sugars may get dangerously high. Check with your doctor and nutritionist to help you identify the best times to take your medications.

If you give yourself injections at multiple sites, use a "fixed rotation" method. For example, if you give yourself three shots a day, choose one site for the morning, a different site for noontime, and yet another site for the evening. With this method, it's still important to vary the injection point within each injection site. The fixed rotations help decrease day-to-day variations in blood sugars caused by varying rates of insulin absorption.

Timing of injections. You'll need to be very consistent with giving yourself the short-acting insulin injections, which are taken at mealtimes. It is important that the insulin enters the bloodstream as glucose levels rise from your consuming food.

The precise timing of the long-acting insulin injections is not as important, although strive to inject yourself at about the same time each day. The exception to this is if you are taking the long-acting insulin called NPH, in which case you will need to be more sensitive to a time schedule. Unlike other long-acting insulin medications, NPH has a peak effect about nine to ten hours after injection. If you are injecting twice a day, you need to give yourself one injection with breakfast and a second injection with either your evening meal or at bedtime. The bedtime dose is preferred because it allows for the peak effect of the insulin to occur as you are getting out of bed the next morning. The concern about giving the injection before your evening meal is that the peak effect of the insulin may occur in the middle of night and lead to low blood sugars.

Storage of insulin. Insulin degrades in the presence of extreme heat, cold, or direct sunlight. It should be kept safely stored in a place where the temperature doesn't vary, such as a refrigerator. The American Diabetes Association (ADA) reports that if you find injecting cold insulin uncomfortable, it is usually safe to store insulin at room temperature for about a month. If you work outdoors, you will need to find a place to store your insulin, or purchase a special insulated storage container to keep with you.

Disposal of needles. Used needles are considered a biological hazard because they may carry diseases that can be transmitted by blood. In some cities, it is illegal to throw loose needles in the trash—it puts others at risk for an accidental stick. Needles must be disposed of in a responsible way. Consider purchasing "sharps containers" made specifically for used needles; these are available in most pharmacies. If you don't have access to a sharps container, drop the needles into a hard plastic bottle and dispose of the bottle. Also, you can ask your healthcare provider for guidelines on the safe disposal of used needles.

Precautions for travel. It's always a good idea to check in with your doctor before traveling to make sure your blood glucose levels are on target. Within the continental United States, most pharmacies will approve your local doctor's request to replace a broken vial or a lost prescription. However, if you are traveling out of the country, take extra vials of insulin in case of breakage. Make sure your insulin is stored at safe temperatures when you travel. If your travel will take you into different time zones that will affect your mealtimes and medication times, you may need to monitor your blood sugars more frequently.

Other Drugs You May Need

If you have type 2 diabetes, you may be at an increased risk for other health problems. These include problems such as high blood pressure, cardiovascular disease, and abnormal cholesterol levels. Accordingly, your doctor may also prescribe other drug therapies.

Blood pressure medications. High blood pressure is a health concern because it raises your chance for heart attack, stroke, and kidney disease. Taking blood pressure medications will help you avoid these health problems.

The drugs most commonly used to control blood pressure in diabetics are *angiotensin receptor blockers* (*ARBs*) and *angiotensin-converting enzyme* (*ACE*) *inhibitors*. These drugs help control blood pressure and also protect against both kidney problems and eye problems associated with diabetes. They are generally used interchangeably, but some people may develop a cough as a side effect from ACE inhibitors. If this happens, your doctor can switch you to an ARB.

Cholesterol medications. High cholesterol levels contribute to cardiovascular disease. Type 2 diabetes further increases the risk of heart disease. As a result, your doctor will likely prescribe a cholesterol-lowering medication.

Drugs that help control cholesterol levels are called *statins*. The ADA recommends that *all* people with type 2 diabetes take a statin (with the exception of women of childbearing age who plan to become pregnant).

Anti-platelet medications. One of the complications associated with cardiovascular disease is blood clots, caused by blood platelets, that become trapped in narrowed blood vessels. Therefore, the ADA recommends a regimen of a daily low-dose aspirin for all individuals with type 2 diabetes over the age of forty. Aspirin acts as a blood thinner and reduces the chances of clot forming.

A Final Note about Medications

Whether you take oral diabetes medications or insulin injections, the medications available today can be very effective, along with diet and exercise, in helping you control blood sugars and preventing long-term complications. It is common to need additional medications or a different type of medication over the course of your treatment. Routine monitoring of your blood glucose and scheduling regular medical checkups will make it possible for your physician to adjust your medications if needed—all in an effort to keep you at optimal health.

You are your own best health advocate. Don't hesitate to ask your healthcare provider questions about any of the medications you're taking.

Rule 6

Avoid Complications by Practicing Good Self-Care

In previous chapters, we discussed how to stay healthy with type 2 diabetes—eat right, exercise, control weight, and take prescribed medications as directed. In this final chapter, we'll discuss the complications that may develop if blood sugar levels are not controlled.

Two major factors contribute to diabetic complications. They are high glucose levels and the length of time the blood sugars have been uncontrolled. The longer blood sugar levels have been uncontrolled, the greater the risk for complications. High blood sugars can damage the walls of blood vessels. Damaged vessels cannot adequately deliver blood to tissues. As a result, tissues are injured—nerves and organs begin losing their ability to function efficiently.

When Are Complications Likely to Occur?

One of the questions most commonly asked by patients with type 2 diabetes is, "How long does it take to develop complications?" There is no single answer for everyone. Your risk of developing complications from diabetes is contingent on a variety of factors, including glucose control, heredity, lifestyle choices, and whether or not you've experienced any complications already.

Some health professionals say complications may show up after ten years of having uncontrolled blood sugars. If you have had type 2 diabetes for some time, but had not been diagnosed until recently, it's difficult to pinpoint how long you may have had the disease, so it's impossible to tell how long it may take to develop complications. If you develop one complication, there's a likelihood that others will follow. For example, when kidney damage occurs, eye problems may develop, too, because both conditions are caused by damage to similar types of small blood vessels.

The good news is that complications can often be prevented, delayed, or sometimes even reversed by controlling blood sugar levels. Clinical studies show that people who lose weight after developing diabetes often return to normal blood sugars. As a result, they can prevent complications.

Types of Complications

Complications of type 2 diabetes are divided into two categories: large blood vessel disease and small blood vessel disease. Large vessel disease causes heart attack, stroke, and *peripheral vascular disease*. Also referred to as *peripheral artery disease* (*PAD*), peripheral vascular disease is a condition in which the arteries that carry blood to the arms or legs become narrowed or clogged. This interferes with the normal flow of blood. When decreased blood flow and infection occurs, amputation of the affected limb may be necessary. Diabetes complications are the most common reason for amputations.

Small vessel disease, as the name suggests, damages the body's small, specialized vessels that serve the eyes, kidneys, and nerves, which are involved in many bodily functions. Damage to these nerves is called *neuropathy*, and there are several forms, depending on the tissues affected.

Peripheral Neuropathy

The most common type of nerve damage caused by type 2 diabetes is *peripheral neuropathy*. It is caused by damage to the delicate coating around the nerves that go to the toes, feet, legs, arms, or hands. Symptoms may include numbness, burning sensations, pain, tingling sensations, sensitivity to touch, muscle weakness, and foot problems such as foot ulcers, infections, or joint and bone pain. These symptoms are often worse at night.

There is no cure for peripheral neuropathy. The best way to prevent this type of nerve damage is to control blood sugars. Even when neuropathy is already present, blood glucose control can help slow the progression of the disease. If you suffer from pain, your doctor may prescribe oral medications or lidocaine patches that are applied to the painful area; the skin absorbs the painkilling medication. Other medications, such as antidepressants, may relieve pain by interfering with signals in the brain that allow you to feel pain. Also, some antiseizure medications may help relieve nerve pain.

This type of neuropathy pain will sometimes diminish, and it's not uncommon to think the condition has improved. However, the decrease in pain may actually result when the nerves have been destroyed, which indicates the neuropathy has actually progressed.

Proximal Neuropathy

The second most common form of diabetic neuropathy, *proximal neuropathy*, causes muscle weakness. It often starts with pain on one side of the body—in the thighs, hips, buttocks, or legs. This type of neuropathy can cause nerve pain that shoots from the lower back down to the legs. These symptoms will usually diminish within a few weeks, depending on the type of nerve damage. Doctors may treat this pain with oral medications. In some cases, physical therapy can help maintain muscle strength until remission occurs.

Autonomic Neuropathy

Autonomic neuropathy refers to damage to the body's autonomic nervous system. The body uses this system of nerves to send messages to and from the brain and spinal cord and to all other parts of the body. These nerves regulate many body functions, including those that involve heart function, eyes, digestive system, urinary tract, sexual function, glucose levels, and perspiration.

Heart Function

Heart function depends in part on the autonomic nervous system. These nerves send signals that accelerate and slow the heart rate, constrict blood vessels, and raise blood pressure. They also control the flow of air into the lungs. When damage occurs to these nerves, the condition is known as *cardiac neuropathy.* Increased heart rate is often one of the first symptoms; irregular heartbeat is another symptom. Some people experience changes in blood pressure; they may have swings in blood pressure levels or experience dizziness or fainting when moving from a sitting to a standing position.

This heart condition, which may progress over time, may be treated with diet and oral medications called beta blockers that prevent the heart rate from becoming elevated and putting a patient at risk for sudden death.

Eye Disease

Diabetic retinopathy is an eye disease that causes damage to the blood vessels in the retina, the thin layer of cells at the back of the eyeball. This is where light is converted into signals and sent to the brain, which, in turn, tells us what we are seeing.

In some cases, tiny blood vessels may swell and leak fluid. In other cases, abnormal blood vessels grow on the surface of the retina. As the disease progresses, you may have blurred vision or see "floaters" on the surface of your eyes. Both eyes are usually affected.

Retinopathy is the most common type of eye disease in people with diabetes and is the most common cause of blindness in American adults under the age of sixty. For this reason, the need for routine eye exams cannot be overstated if you have type 2 diabetes. Retinopathy can sneak up on you, because often there are no symptoms until permanent tissue damage has occurred. However, if it is diagnosed early, there is a good chance the disease can be successfully treated.

Consistent blood sugar and blood pressure control can prevent or decrease retinopathy's progression. Another treatment option is laser surgery, in which a laser beam stops vessels from leaking. Newer forms of treatment involve injecting steroids into the back of the eyeball and therapies that inhibit the leaking of fluid into the retina.

Digestive System

When nerves involving the stomach are affected, it can cause a condition called *gastroparesis*, which inhibits food from being digested normally. Symptoms may include heartburn, abdominal pain, feeling full for prolonged periods after a meal, and vomiting. Gastroparesis can also make blood glucose levels fluctuate as the result of poor food digestion. Severe cases can lead to nausea, vomiting, bloating, and loss of appetite. Treatments may include medications, changes in eating habits, and changes in diabetes medications. More advanced cases may require a feeding tube or the implantation of a device that sends electrical pulses to control nausea and vomiting.

When nerves related to bowel functioning are damaged, constipation or diarrhea may occur. If nerves to the esophagus are damaged, swallowing problems may develop. Medications may help with some of these intestinal problems.

Urinary Tract

Autonomic neuropathy may affect the body's nerves involved in urination. Damage to these nerves may affect a person's ability to sense that the bladder is full; this can lead to incontinence. Also, the bladder may not empty completely, which can lead to urinary tract infections.

Kidney disease caused by diabetes, also known as *nephropathy*, occurs when tiny blood vessels in the kidney are damaged. The kidneys are not able to filter and control the excretion of urine. Kidney failure occurs if the kidneys stop working altogether.

There are no early symptoms of kidney disease; however, physicians can determine how well kidneys are functioning by performing a test on a urine sample for the presence of *albumin,* a protein that does not normally leak into the urine. When it does leak, this can be one of the earliest signs of diabetes-related kidney disease.

The best way to prevent kidney disease is the early management of glucose levels and blood pressure, which can also affect kidney function. Regular screening for kidney disease is important since early detection and medications can prevent the progression of this disease.

The use of drugs called ACE inhibitors and ARBs, which lower blood pressure, have been shown to decrease albumin excretion in the urine and protect kidney function. One of these drugs may also be prescribed if you have high blood pressure.

If the kidney disease is severe when diagnosed, aggressively controlling blood sugar, blood pressure, and lipid levels are the only effective methods to prevent further decline. Over-the-counter and prescription nonsteroidal, anti-inflammatory medications are typically not recommended for kidney problems.

Sexual Function

Autonomic neuropathy in men may cause erectile dysfunction. In order for a man to have an erection, his brain must be able to send signals from his spinal cord to his penis. If nerves are damaged, the signal may not be received, and the erection does not occur.

To avoid diabetes-related male sexual dysfunction, maintain blood sugar control, stop smoking, and avoid excessive alcohol intake. Treating the diabetes may help restore potency. Other treatments in the form of prescription medication and self-administered injections may be helpful. Results vary based on the severity of the nerve

Reduce Your Risk for Complications

You can reduce the risk of diabetes complications. For every 1 percent reduction in the hemoglobin A1c level, type 2 diabetes patients reduce their risk of developing eye, kidney, and nerve disease by 40 percent.

Source: Centers for Disease Control and Prevention

damage. Surgery to insert penile implants is another option. If a low libido persists after making these changes, consider having your doctor check your testosterone level. Testosterone replacement therapy may be an option.

In women, nerve damage may lead to lack of sexual arousal, and difficulty with lubrication and orgasm. Bringing blood sugar levels under control may alleviate these symptoms. Treatments may involve topical creams or hormone therapy.

For some women with diabetes, getting pregnant is a challenge. Poor blood sugar control can lead to irregular menstrual cycles and difficulty conceiving. Lowering blood sugar levels and taking diabetes medications along with fertility medications often improve the chances of conception.

A woman's ability to safely become pregnant and carry a child to term depends on her health over the years prior to conception. Complications, including retinopathy and nephropathy, can rapidly progress in women who are pregnant and have diabetes.

Lack of Awareness of Low Blood Sugars

Blood sugar levels are considered too low if they drop below 70 mg/dl. If you've ever had a drop in your blood sugars, you know the symptoms—weakness, shakiness, hunger, and sweating. However, nerve damage can also prevent you from feeling the usual warning signs; you remain unaware that your blood sugar levels have dropped below normal. This condition is called *hypoglycemia unawareness*. Even though you may not experience the usual symptoms of low blood sugars, you may feel irritable or even irrational.

Hypoglycemia unawareness is more common among people with type 1 diabetes and those who have had type 2 diabetes for a number of years.

In this situation, frequent blood testing is the best way to be aware of drops in blood sugar levels. When levels are low, you can take actions to raise your blood sugars. If left untreated, and blood sugars drop too low, you may lose consciousness. Immediate, emergency medical treatment is needed since this condition can be life-threatening. For this reason, patients are prescribed *glucagon,* a hormone that reverses the low blood sugars, to be given by family or friends when the patient is unable to take oral glucose to reverse the reaction.

Perspiration

Autonomic nerve damage may affect the body's ability to control its temperature. As a result, you do not perspire norm-ally. Symptoms may include heavy night sweating. Symptoms may also include the inability to sweat, especially in the legs and feet. In some people, certain foods, often cheese, will cause sweating.

Focal Neuropathy

The types of neuropathy we've discussed so far involve multiple nerves. However, *focal neuropathy* involves, or focuses on, just a single nerve. The symptoms depend on which nerve is affected; it may be a nerve that affects the head, the torso, or the leg. When symptoms affect the head, it can cause eye problems; you may have double vision, pain behind the eye, or problems with focusing; paralysis on one side of the face, called Bell's palsy, may also occur.

Symptoms in the torso may include pain in the lower back, chest, side, or abdomen. Other symptoms may cause pain in the thigh, shin, or foot.

This type of neuropathy can also cause what's called *nerve compression.* Carpal tunnel syndrome is the most common example. Symptoms include numbness, tingling, or weakness in the hands and fingers.

Focal neuropathy often comes on suddenly and typically affects older adults. Fortunately, however, the symptoms usually improve over a period of a few weeks or months, and no permanent damage occurs.

Improvement in blood sugar control decreases pain caused by focal neuropathy. Oral medications can be used for pain that does not respond to glucose control.

Diabetes Neuropathies

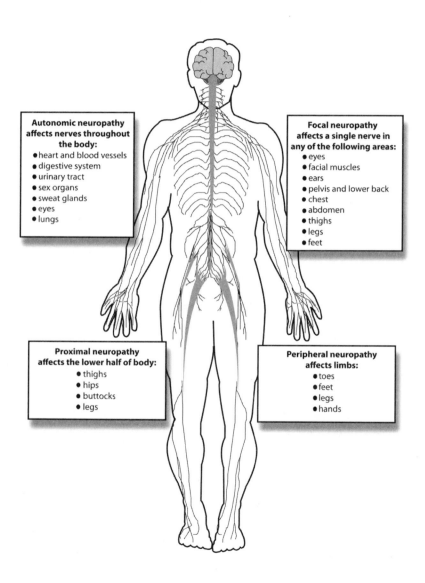

Autonomic neuropathy affects nerves throughout the body:
- heart and blood vessels
- digestive system
- urinary tract
- sex organs
- sweat glands
- eyes
- lungs

Focal neuropathy affects a single nerve in any of the following areas:
- eyes
- facial muscles
- ears
- pelvis and lower back
- chest
- abdomen
- thighs
- legs
- feet

Proximal neuropathy affects the lower half of body:
- thighs
- hips
- buttocks
- legs

Peripheral neuropathy affects limbs:
- toes
- feet
- legs
- hands

Heart Disease

We've discussed how damage to small blood vessels can cause injury to nerves that affect heart function. However, other forms of cardiovascular disease occur as the result of damage to the body's large blood vessels. These cardiovascular diseases include: atherosclerosis, stroke, and peripheral vascular disease.

Atherosclerosis

How does damage occur in large blood vessels? Healthy coronary arteries have smooth, flexible walls that deliver blood to the heart. However, over many years, these flexible walls can become progressively irritated and clogged by *plaque*, which includes such substances as fats, cholesterol, calcium, and cellular debris. When these arteries become narrowed, you're said to have a form of coronary heart disease called *atherosclerosis*. High blood sugars contribute to this disease; other contributing factors include: high LDL cholesterol, high triglycerides, low HDL cholesterol, high blood pressure, and smoking.

If the blood vessels become too clogged, a heart attack can occur. Common symptoms of heart attack include:

- uncomfortable pressure, tightness, fullness, squeezing, or pain in the center of the chest
- pain that lasts more than a few minutes (thirty minutes to several hours) or goes away and comes back
- pain that spreads to the shoulders, neck, or arms
- light-headedness or fainting
- nausea
- profuse sweating
- shortness of breath

A heart attack is a medical emergency. If you or someone else is experiencing these symptoms, call 911 immediately and say someone is having a heart attack. Patients receive help immediately upon arrival by paramedics, and are transported to a hospital by ambulance. Patients reach a hospital sooner in an ambulance than if they are taken by friends or relatives.

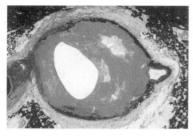 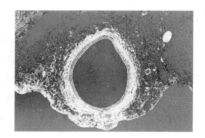

Blocked artery. Plaque buildup obstructs the flow of blood through this artery. The white area in the center is the only portion of the artery not blocked.

Normal Artery. An open artery easily transports oxygenated blood away from the heart and to other parts of the body. *Custom Medical Stock Photo, Inc.*

Stroke

A stroke is a "brain attack" in the same way the blockage of blood flow to the heart is a heart attack. A stroke occurs when an area of the brain is deprived of blood flow. The leading cause of stroke is a *thrombosis,* or blood clot. Clots develop gradually when the inner lining of blood vessels become clogged with the buildup of cholesterol and fatty substances. Symptoms of a stroke include:

- sudden numbness or weakness of the face, arm, or leg, especially on one side of the body
- sudden confusion, trouble speaking or understanding
- sudden trouble seeing in one or both eyes
- sudden trouble walking, dizziness, loss or balance or coordination
- sudden, severe headache with no known cause

Like a heart attack, a stroke is a medical emergency. Treatment will start sooner by calling 911 and asking for an ambulance.

Peripheral Vascular Disease

As mentioned earlier, peripheral vascular disease (also called peripheral artery disease) occurs when fatty deposits narrow blood vessels in the legs, and circulation to the legs and feet is impaired. Symptoms may include:

- leg pain when walking (pain may stop after resting)
- numbness, tingling, or coldness in the lower legs or feet
- discoloration of tissues in the legs or feet
- sores on the feet that are slow to heal

Peripheral vascular disease is associated with an increased risk of heart attack and stroke.

Preventing Cardiovascular Risks

If you're at risk for heart disease, stroke, or peripheral vascular disease, it's important to lower blood sugars, blood pressure, and cholesterol levels, and stop smoking. Exercise is important; physical activity actually repairs blood vessel walls and makes them healthier. Weight loss, especially losing abdominal fat, is important since these fat tissues can release acids and hormones that make insulin resistance worse.

Specific guidelines for reducing the risk of heart attack, stroke, and peripheral arterial disease include: maintain a hemoglobin A1c level below 7 percent; keep blood pressure lower than 130/80; aim for an LDL cholesterol level of 100 mg/dl or less.

If you have already suffered a heart attack or a stroke or you are over forty years old, your doctor may prescribe a daily, low-dose aspirin. Aspirin thins the blood and reduces the chances of blood clots forming. Your physician may put you on an aggressive cholesterol-lowering medication, as well.

Other Complications
Risk of Infection

High blood sugar levels inhibit our body's ability to fight off infection. Because elevated blood glucose can decrease blood flow, the body has a decreased ability to repair tissues, and bacterial infections can result. Areas of numbness, caused

Reminders for Sick Days

Contact your healthcare provider if:

- you feel too sick to eat normally and are unable to keep down food over a 6-hour period
- you're having severe diarrhea
- you lose 5 pounds or more
- your temperature is over 101 degrees F
- your blood glucose is lower than 70 or remains over 300 mg/dl
- you're having trouble breathing
- you feel sleepy or can't think clearly

If you feel sleepy or can't think clearly, have someone call your healthcare provider or take you to an emergency room.

Source: Centers for Disease Control and Prevention

by nerve damage, are breeding grounds for infection because you may not be able to feel the pain of the injury and react to the injury in a timely fashion. For this reason, it is imperative that you check your skin frequently for any sores or signs of infection.

Taking simple precautionary measures can prevent serious problems in the future. Pay special attention to checking your feet. Because feet are less visible than other body parts, sores or injuries may go unnoticed. Examine your feet daily if you have decreased sensation in them; it's important to protect the skin from cuts or injury that could lead to infections.

Wear comfortable shoes that don't cause blisters or calluses. Try shoes with inserts designed to disperse pressure on the foot. This prevents putting too much pressure on any one part of your foot and decreases your risk of developing a foot ulcer. If you do find blisters or calluses, have them removed promptly or ask a healthcare professional for guidance on how to treat them. You also may consider getting screened by a healthcare professional for a pre-ulcer condition. This screening involves a thorough exam and being asked questions about previous foot problems. Based on the exam, a healthcare professional can assess your risk for complications involving the feet.

If you develop an infection in either of your feet (or any body part), treatment consists of blood sugar control and antibiotic therapy. Most severe infections respond to a combi-

Things to Do At Least Once a Year

- Get a dilated-eye exam.
- Get a foot exam, including check of circulation and nerves.
- Get a flu shot in October to mid-November.
- Get a pneumonia shot as directed by your doctor.
- Get your blood pressure checked.
- Get a kidney test:
  - ✓ Have your urine tested for albumin.
  - ✓ Have your blood tested for chemicals that measure kidney function.
- Get your blood fats checked for:
  - ✓ Total cholesterol.
  - ✓ High-density lipoprotein (HDL).
  - ✓ Low-density lipoprotein (LDL).
  - ✓ Triglycerides.
- Get a dental exam at least twice a year.
- Talk with your healthcare team about:
  - ✓ How well you can sense low blood glucose.
  - ✓ How you are treating high blood glucose.
  - ✓ Tobacco use (cigarettes, cigars, pipes, smokeless tobacco).
  - ✓ Your feelings about having diabetes.
  - ✓ Your plans for pregnancy if you're a woman.

Source: Centers for Disease Control and Prevention

nation of alleviating pressure on the affected area, aggressive wound healing, antibiotics, removal of dead skin, and an aggressive follow-up regimen. Amputation occurs only in extreme cases and is a last resort.

Skin Complications

People with diabetes may experience a variety of skin problems. One of the most common skin complications is neuropathy-induced ulcers. Ulcers are created when too much pressure is put on one spot; however, the nerve damage may prevent you from feeling the pressure, and the tissue can become injured. Preventive measures include avoiding any points of excessive pressure on your body.

Diabetic shin spots are another skin condition that may develop in people with diabetes. These spots occur on the shins after minor scrapes or injury. They may develop into discolored lesions and remain for prolonged periods of time. Protecting your shins from injury prevents the skin in these areas from breaking down.

Another common skin disorder among those who take insulin injections is a condition called *lipohypertrophy*. It results from insulin being injected at the same site repeatedly over time. The repeated injections may cause an accumulation of fat under the skin. This lump may be unsightly, mildly painful, and permanent. Continued insulin injections at this site may result in poor insulin absorption and erratic blood sugars.

Anyone with diabetes is at greater risk for fungal infections, especially in the toenails and feet. High blood sugars can cause skin to become inflamed and infected. Nails affected by a fungal infection become thicker and darker and are sometimes quite disfiguring. This condition is often difficult to treat. Oral treatments can be toxic to the liver, and topical ointments are often not effective.

Gum Disease

Gum disease is a breakdown of the normal gum structures within the mouth, often leading to tooth loss and infection. Poor blood sugar control increases the risk of *periodontitis*, an infection to the skin around the teeth; it can lead to pockets of inflammation that can cause tooth loss or abscess formation. Sore, swollen, or inflamed gums that bleed when you brush are symptoms of another condition called *gingivitis*. Like other infections, these dental diseases can cause blood glucose levels to rise.

Gum disease is commonly treated with a combination of antibiotics, routine brushing, and using an antiseptic mouthwash to kill germs. In severe cases, teeth may need to be pulled. Gum disease is usually preventable with routine dental care.

Complications in Pregnancy

Pregnant women who have type 2 diabetes may be at risk for having a baby with birth defects, so it is essential to have blood sugars under control before becoming pregnant. Studies have demonstrated that the higher the woman's hemoglobin A1c level during pregnancy, the greater the risks are to both her and the fetus.

Other potential complications in pregnant women with diabetes include eye disease in the mother, premature birth, high birth weight, and even fetal death, which may result from poor blood flow to the uterus. The mother is also at risk for *toxemia*, a dangerously elevated blood pressure, during pregnancy. In cases of severe toxemia, delivery may be induced prematurely to save a woman's life, but may jeopardize the life of her baby.

If you are a woman with type 2 diabetes, it's important to plan your pregnancy carefully. Ask your physician to assess your potential for complications prior to conception. You want to be able to safely sustain the physical changes that come with pregnancy. If your blood glucose is under control when you become pregnant, there is a good chance that, with proper medical care, your pregnancy will proceed without complications.

When You Are Sick

Being sick when you have type 2 diabetes means you'll need to take a few extra precautions. Blood sugars can fluctuate when you are ill. For example, having the flu may make your glucose levels rise. Further, the flu may impair your immune system so that you may become much sicker. Infections will increase glucose levels.

Sometimes when you're ill, you may not feel like eating. But, as you already know, your food intake, or lack of it, can affect blood sugars. Do not stop taking your diabetes medications. If you are not able to eat or keep food down, contact your healthcare professional about how to ensure that you receive enough carbohydrates to nourish your body and help you maintain glucose levels. Check your blood sugars more frequently, making sure levels are not too high or too low.

Tips for Good Self-Care

Throughout this book, we have discussed the lifestyle changes that will help you successfully manage type 2 diabetes and move on with living a healthier life. Good self-care starts with learning about type 2 diabetes and learning how to control your blood sugars. Consider taking a class taught by a diabetes education professional. Your physician can refer you to an educator. These professionals can offer guidance that will become a foundation for your plan of good self-care.

Here's a review of the guidelines for making changes that will influence your health for years to come.

Consistently monitor and control blood glucose levels. It is imperative that you check your blood sugars regularly at home to ensure that you are maintaining your target glucose level. Keeping glucose levels under control is crucial to avoiding complications.

Eat nutritiously. Choosing a healthful diet is one of the most important things you can do to manage type 2 diabetes. It helps you keep blood sugars within normal ranges and promotes weight loss. Fad diets rarely work. Choose an eating plan that you can live with as part of a permanent lifestyle plan.

Maintain your target weight. Being overweight not only contributes to insulin resistance, it also causes diabetes medications to not work as well. If you need to lose weight, aim for losing one to two pounds per week. A healthy weight will make your treatment of diabetes more successful overall.

Exercise regularly. Like good nutrition, regular exercise is crucial for managing type 2 diabetes. Exercised muscles are more likely to respond well to insulin. Be patient with yourself in setting up an exercise plan. Don't try jogging for 30 minutes the first week of an exercise program. The keys to success are to start slowly, increase the effort gradually, and do it consistently. Aim for 150 minutes of moderate intensity exercise weekly.

Quit smoking. Smoking aggravates blood vessel abnormalities. The combination of diabetes and smoking is especially damaging. If you are a smoker, talk to your physician about the best method for you to quit.

Check your feet for sores. Examining your feet regularly will help you identify and care for any wounds that could lead to infection. Wash your feet daily and dry them well, especially between the toes. Moisture promotes the growth of bacteria. Don't soak your feet—this causes dryness. Trim toenails after bathing, when the nails are softer. Do not cut away corns or calluses, and don't use liquid corn or callous removers since they can damage skin tissue. Talk to your doctor about how to use a pumice stone to gently rub away corns and callouses. Using lotion on your feet will prevent skin from becoming dry and cracked, which makes it an entry point for bacteria.

Always wear shoes and clean socks that are made of cotton or wool, which helps keep feet dry. To avoid injury, never go barefoot, even inside your house.

See your physician for regular checkups. If your diabetes is well controlled, you may need to be examined by your doctor only twice a year. If you are having problems controlling your diabetes, however, see your physician every three months. During your exam, you and your doctor can discuss your treatment goals, any adjustments needed for medications, and whether you need to make additional lifestyle changes.

When you visit your physician, take your glucose testing log. Your doctor can see whether your levels are consistently within target ranges. Some patients feel ashamed to show their doctors their glucose logs if their levels are outside target ranges. However, it is essential that you are honest with your healthcare provider. Your doctor's intent is not to judge you, but rather to deliver the best possible treatment. When it comes to recording blood sugar levels, it's also important to be honest with yourself.

Get regular eye exams. Those who develop eye complications often have no warnings or changes in eyesight. Your optometrist or eye physician should screen for eye complications once a year. During your exam, your doctor will dilate your eyes to check for any leaking or bleeding in the blood vessels. Early diagnosis of this complication may prevent further problems and lead to more-successful treatment.

Visit your dentist twice a year. Your dentist will monitor any inflammation in your gums. Regular teeth cleaning and daily hygiene can prevent gum disease. Brush and floss your teeth at least twice a day, including at bedtime. Use a soft-bristle brush and replace it every few months.

In Closing

Unlike so many other diseases, you can control type 2 diabetes with lifestyle changes and medications. Complications can often be prevented, delayed, or sometimes even reversed by keeping tight controls on blood sugar levels. Clinical studies show that people who lose weight after developing diabetes have a return to normal blood sugars. As a result, they can prevent complications.

You have the power to stay healthy with type 2 diabetes. However, you don't need to make all the changes alone. Your chances for success will improve significantly if you have support. Ask for help from physicians, nurses, dieticians, diabetes educators, and from family and friends. Abundant amounts of help and support are available. Ask for help. You deserve it.

Appendix

Meal Plan • 1400-1500 Calories

Breakfast – 3 carb servings (45g)	**Carbohydrates**
2 slices whole wheat toast	30 grams
½ grapefruit	15 grams
1 poached egg	0 grams
1 T. light margarine	0 grams

Lunch – 3 carb servings (45g)	
1 cup vegetable soup	15 grams
6 saltine crackers	15 grams
¾ cup cottage cheese	0 grams
15 grapes	15 grams

Afternoon snack – 1 carb serving (15g)	
6 oz. light yogurt	18 grams

Dinner – 4 carb servings (60g)	
3-5 oz. baked fish	0 grams
1 medium baked potato (6 oz.)	30 grams
1 5-inch ear corn on the cob	15 grams
1 cup melon cubes	15 grams
large lettuce salad	0-5 grams
1 T. light margarine (50 calories per T.)	0 grams
2 T. light dressing	0-5 grams

Evening snack – 1 carb serving (15g)	
3 cups light popcorn	15 grams

Reprinted with permission from Nebraska Medical Center Diabetes Center

Meal Plan • 1650-1800 Calories

Breakfast – 4 carb servings (45g)	**Carbohydrates**
1 cup 1% milk	12 grams
1 cup bran flakes	30 grams
½ banana	15 grams

Lunch – 4 carb servings (45g)

2 slices whole wheat bread	30 grams
2-3 oz. lean turkey breast	0 grams
1-2 tsp. mustard or light mayonnaise	0 grams
1 cup vegetable soup	15 grams
15 grapes	15 grams
relishes	5 grams

Afternoon snack – 1 carb serving (15g)

3 cups light popcorn	15 grams

Dinner – 4 carb servings (60g)

3 oz. lean roast beef	0 grams
1 medium baked potato (6 oz.)	30 grams
¾ cup pineapple	23 grams
lettuce salad	0-1 grams
1 cup green beans	5-10 grams
1 T. light margarine (50 calories per T.)	0 grams

Evening snack – 1 carb serving (15g)

1 orange	15 grams

Meal Plan • 1650-1800 Calories

Breakfast – 4 carb servings (60g)   **Carbohydrates**

2 slices whole wheat toast	30 grams
1-2 poached eggs	0 grams
1 slice crisp bacon or ½ oz. ham	0 grams
1 T. diet margarine	0 grams

Lunch – 4 carb servings (60g)

small roast beef sandwich	33 grams
garden salad	12 grams
2 T. reduced calorie dressing	3 grams
1 small apple	15 grams

Afternoon snack – 1 carb serving (15g)

15 grapes	15 grams

Dinner – 4 carb servings (60g)

3-5 oz. baked fish	0 grams
1 cup rice	45 grams
½ cup peas	15 grams
lettuce salad w/ raw vegetables	0-5 grams
1-2 T. salad dressing	0-5 grams

Evening snack – 1 carb serving (15g)

½ cup sugar-free chocolate pudding	15 grams

Meal Plan • 1650-1800 Calories

Breakfast – 4 carb servings (60g)   Carbohydrates

1 cup cream of wheat	30 grams
1 slice whole wheat toast	15 grams
½ cup 1% milk	6 grams
½ cup raspberries	8 grams
1 tsp. light margarine	0 grams

Lunch – 4 carb servings (60g)

2 slices whole wheat bread	30 grams
3-5 oz. lean meat	0 grams
½ cup chicken noodle soup	15 grams
2 saltine crackers	5 grams
1 cup cooked carrots	10 grams
relish	0-5 grams
1-2 tsp. light mayonnaise or mustard	0 grams

Afternoon snack – 1 carb serving (15g)

1 small pear	15 grams

Dinner – 4 carb servings (60g)

3-4 oz. ground beef in sauce	0 grams
1 cup pasta	30 grams
½ cup light spaghetti sauce	8 grams
2 small pieces Italian bread	20 grams
lettuce salad w/ raw vegetables	0-5 grams
1-2 T. salad dressing	0-5 grams

Evening snack – 1 carb serving (15g)

½ cup 1% cottage cheese	3 grams
½ cup canned "lite" peaches	15 grams

Meal Plan • 1650-1800 Calories

Breakfast – 4 carb servings (60g)

	Carbohydrates
1 whole English muffin	30 grams
½ grapefruit	15 grams
1 T. diet margarine	0 grams
2 tsp. jam	9 grams

Lunch – 4 carb servings (60g)

| Chicken, steak or veggie fajita wrap | 50-53 grams |
| ¾ cup strawberries | 8-10 grams |

Afternoon snack – 1 carb serving (15g)

| 1 granola bar | 20 grams |

Dinner – 4 carb servings (60g)

2 grilled pork chops	0 grams
1 small baked potato (3 oz.)	15 grams
2 small ears corn on the cob	30 grams
1 medium tomato, sliced	5 grams
1 cup watermelon cubes	10 grams

Evening snack – 1 carb serving (15g)

| ½ cup "lite" ice cream | 15 grams |

Meal Plan • 1800-1900 Calories

Breakfast – 4 carb servings (60g)

Carbohydrates

½ cup cereal	22 grams
½ cup skim milk	6 grams
2 slices whole wheat toast	30 grams
1 T. light margarine	0 grams

Lunch – 4 carb servings (60g)

turkey sandwich:

2 slices whole wheat bread	30 grams
2-3 oz. shaved turkey	0 grams
1 oz. fat-free cheese	2 grams
1 medium tomato	5 grams
onion, mustard	0 grams
1 small apple	15 grams

Afternoon snack – 1 ½ carb servings (22g)

Low-fat granola bar	22 grams

Dinner – 5 carb servings (75g)

2 small, lean pork chops	0 grams
2/3 cup pork n' beans	30 grams
1 small blueberry muffin	30 grams
2 T. light dressing	0-5 grams
1 ¼ cup strawberries w/ sugar-free sweetener	15 grams
1-2 T. fat-free whipped topping	2 grams

Evening snack – 1 carb serving (15g)

3 cups light popcorn	15 grams

Glossary

alpha-glucosidase inhibitors: Oral drugs that slow the rate at which glucose (sugars) are absorbed by the intestines

angiotensin-converting enzyme (ACE) inhibitors: Medications that enlarge blood vessels, reducing blood pressure

angiotensin receptor blockers (ARBs): Medications that enlarge the blood vessels by blocking chemicals that cause muscles to constrict and press on blood vessels

atherosclerosis: Also often known as "hardening of the arteries," this condition is caused by collection of fatty material (plaque) inside artery walls

autonomic neuropathy: A group of symptoms, not a specific disease, that results from damage to the nervous system

basal insulin: The amount of insulin needed to regulate changes in the body's daily blood sugar levels

biguanides: Medications that regulate the way the body manages insulin

bolus insulin: Rapid-working injected insulin that helps the body manage a rise in blood sugar levels caused by a meal

cardiac autonomic neuropathy (CAN): Damage to the nerves in the heart that can lead to changes in blood pressure as well as heart rate

cortisol: Also called hydrocortisone, a steroid hormone normally produced by the adrenal gland in reaction to stress

diabetic retinopathy: Damage to blood vessels in the eye's retina

diastolic pressure: Blood pressure when the heart is resting

DPP-4 inhibitors: Medications that decrease blood sugars, increase insulin, and enhance the body's own ability to lower blood sugar

duration (of insulin): Length of time insulin is active measured in terms of onset, peak effect, and duration of action

echocardiogram: Test using sound waves to create a moving picture of the heart

fasting blood glucose test: Blood test measuring of blood sugar levels after a set number of hours without food

focal neuropathy: Nerve damage or inflammation causing pain in a single nerve

gastroparesis: A condition affecting the ability of the stomach to empty; also called "delayed gastric emptying"

gestational diabetes: Diabetes that starts, or is first discovered, during pregnancy

gingivitis: Inflammation of the gums

glucagon: Pancreatic hormone that raises blood sugar

glucometer: Monitoring device that measures blood sugar levels

glucose: Type of sugar that occurs in plants and animals

Hemoglobin A1c test: Blood test that indicates how well the body is metabolizing sugars over time

hyperglycemia: High levels of sugar in the body

hypertension: High blood pressure

hypoglycemia: Low levels of sugar in the body

hypoglycemia unawareness: Sudden severe reaction caused by an unrecognized drop in blood sugar

incretin mimetics: Injectable drugs that lower blood sugar by imitating body hormones

insulin resistance: Condition where the body produces insulin but can't use it properly

Glossary

insulin resistance syndrome: A cluster of abnormalities caused by body tissues' diminished ability to respond to the action of insulin

LDL (low-density lipoprotein): A molecule that is a combination of fat and protein; also called "bad" cholesterol

LDL cholesterol: Molecules that can form plaque in blood vessels; also called "bad" cholesterol

lipohypertrophy: Fatty lump under the skin caused by repeated insulin injections in the same spot

meglitinides: Oral diabetic medications that increase insulin

metabolic syndrome: Name for a group of risk factors that occur together and increase the risk for coronary artery disease, stroke, and type 2 diabetes

metformin: Oral drug used alone, or with insulin, to control blood sugar levels

microalbumin: Protein found in blood plasma and urine that can indicate kidney disease

monounsaturated fats: Type of fat nutrient that lowers total cholesterol and "bad" cholesterol levels while increasing "good" cholesterol levels

nephropathy: Damage to, or disease of, the kidney; also called nephrosis

nerve compression: Nerves trapped, usually near joints subject to inflammation or swelling, that result in muscle weakness or wasting

neuropathy: Any disease or malfunction of nerves or the nervous system

omega-3 fatty acids: Polyunsaturated fats found in many vegetables and fish that reduce cholesterol levels and have anti-inflammatory properties

onset (of insulin): Time it takes for oral or injected insulin to take effect

oral glucose tolerance test: Test that measures the body's ability to use sugar (glucose)

peak time (of insulin): Time when insulin is working its hardest

peridontitis: Gum disease caused by plaque and bacteria spreading and growing below the gum line

peripheral artery disease (PAD): A common circulatory problem in which narrowed arteries reduce blood flow to arms and legs

peripheral neuropathy: Problems with nerves that carry information to and from the brain to the spinal cord, muscles, skin, joints, or internal organs

peripheral vascular disease: Diseases of blood vessels outside the heart and brain that lead to narrowing and hardening of the arteries that supply the legs and feet

polyunsaturated fats: Fats that can lower the level of "bad" cholesterol; they generally remain liquid even at low temperatures

postprandial: After eating

proximal neuropathy: Nerve damage causing pain and weakness in the thighs, hips, buttocks, or legs

random plasma glucose test: A blood test that measures blood sugars without regard to when the person last ate; also called "casual plasma glucose test"

saturated fats: Fats that raise total blood cholesterol as well as "bad" cholesterol and are mainly found in animal products and some fatty vegetable oils

statins: Drugs used to lower cholesterol levels

sulfonylureas: Drugs used to increase insulin production by the pancreas

Syndrome X: Another name for "metabolic syndrome" or "insulin resistance syndrome"

synthetic amylin hormone: Hormone produced by the pancreas that signals the brain that enough food has been eaten and the stomach is "full"

systolic pressure: Blood pressure when the heart is contracting

thiazolidinediones (TZDs): Drugs that help the body better metabolize insulin by increasing sensitivity to its effects

thrombosis: Blood clot formed in a blood vessel

toxemia: A generic term for the presence of toxins in the blood. Also used to describe "preeclampsia," a pregnancy condition in which high blood pressure and protein in the urine develop after the twentieth week of pregnancy

trans fats: Created by adding hydrogen to vegetable oil and often used in food manufacturing, these raise "bad" cholesterol and lower "good" cholesterol

unsaturated fats: Fats that are liquid at ordinary temperatures

Resources

American Association of Diabetes Educators
100 West Monroe, 4th Floor
Chicago, Illinois 60603-1901
Phone: (800) 832-6874
www.diabeteseducator.org

American Diabetes Association
1701 North Beauregard Street
Alexandria, VA 22311
Phone: (800) 342–2383
www.diabetes.org

American Dietetic Association
216 West Jackson Boulevard, Suite 800
Chicago, Illinois 60606-6995
Phone: (800) 745-0775
www.eatright.org

American Heart Association
7272 Greenville Avenue
Dallas, TX 75231
Phone: (800) 242-8721
www.heart.org

Diabetes Exercise and Sports Association
P.O. Box 1935
Litchfield Park, AZ 85340
Phone: (800) 898-4322
www.diabetes-exercise.org

Foundation of the American Academy
of Ophthalmology Diabetes Project
P.O. Box 429098
San Francisco, California 94142-9098
Phone: (800) 222-3937
www.aao.org

Juvenile Diabetes Research
Foundation International
26 Broadway, 14th Floor
New York, NY 10004
Phone: (800) 533–2873
www.jdrf.org

National Diabetes Education Clearinghouse
1 Information Way
Bethesda, Maryland 20892-3560
Phone: (800) 438-5383
www.ndep.nih.gov

National Diabetes Education Program
1 Diabetes Way
Bethesda, MD 20892–3560
Phone: (800) 38–5383
www.ndep.nih.gov

National Eye Institute
2020 Vision Place
Bethesda, MD 20892-3655

Phone: (800) 869-2020
www.nei.nih.gov

National Kidney Foundation
30 East 33rd Street
New York, NY 10016
Phone: (800) 622-9010
www.kidney.org

Index

erectile dysfunction, 83
esophagus, 82
ethnicity, 4
excessive hunger, 5, 63
excessive thirst, 5, 63
exercise, 41–52, 61, 94, 95
    benefits, 41
    safety precautions, 50, 51
exercise program, 45
eye disease, 81, 82
eye examinations, 96

F

fast food, 35
fasting, 7, 8, 57
fasting blood glucose, 10
fasting blood glucose test,
    6, 7, 57
    classifications, 7
fat, 33
fatigue, 5, 63
fiber, 18, 38, 39
flexibility, 44
    exercises, 48
fluid retention, 67
focal neuropathy, 85, 86
    symptoms, 85
Food and Drug
    Administration, 34, 67
food basics, 16–23
food diary, 59
food labels, 31–34
foot ulcers, 80
frequent urination, 5, 63
fungal infections, 92

G

gallbladder, 3
gastrointestinal system, 68
gastroparesis, 82
genetics, 4
gestational diabetes, 4, 6
gingivitis, 92

gluagaon, 85
glucagon-like peptide-1
    (GLP-1), 67
glucometer, 53
glucose, 2, 3, 8
glucose meter, 53
    choosing, 53, 54
    guidelines, 55
    using, 54–56
glucose test results, 57, 59
good fats, 19, 20
gum disease, 92, 93

H

HDL (high-density
    lipoprotein) cholesterol,
    9, 10, 43, 87
headache, 63
heart attack, 1, 12, 15, 20,
    76
    symptoms, 87
heart disease, 42, 87
heart function, 81
heartburn, 67, 82
hemoglobin A1c test, 8, 9,
    60, 93
high blood pressure, 9–12,
    42, 87
high fasting blood glucose,
    9
high triglycerides, 11
hormone, 4, 44, 85
hormone levels, 62
hormone replacement
    therapy (HRT), 62
hormone therapy, 84
hydrogenation, 21
hyperglycemia, 62
    managing, 63
hypertension, 11
hypoglycemia, 22, 62, 64,
    67, 70, 71, 84
    managing, 63

113

neuropathy, 78–96
neuropathy-induced ulcers, 91
non-insulin injections, 69, 70
numbness in hands and feet, 1, 6, 63, 79, 85, 89
nutrition, 14–40
nutritionist, 17

O

obesity, 4, 9
omega-3 fatty acids, 20
oral diabetes medications, 65–69
oral glucose tolerance test, 7, 8
osteoporosis, 67

P

pancreas, 2, 3, 66, 68
periodontitis, 92
peripheral artery disease, 88
peripheral neuropathy, 79, 80, 86
symptoms, 79, 80
peripheral vascular disease, 87–89
personal trainer, 46
perspiration, 85
physical activity, 42
physical inactivity, 4
plaque, 87
platelets, 77
polyunsaturated fats, 20
pregnancy, 4, 76, 93
prescription medications, 62
protein, 19, 33
proximal neuropathy, 80, 86

R

random plasma glucose test, 7
rapid-acting insulin, 71
recommended sources of carbohydrates, 18
recommended sources of fats, 20
recommended sources of protein, 19
recording glucose meter results, 59, 60
red blood cells, 8
resistance training, 47
retesting blood sugar levels, 56
retinopathy, 81, 82, 84

S

saturated fats, 12, 15
sedentary lifestyle, 42
self-care, 78–96
serving size, 32
setting exercise goals, 45
sexual function, 81, 83, 84
shakiness, 63
sharps container, 75
shortness of breath, 87
skin complications, 91, 92
skin rashes, 67
slow-healing wounds, 5, 63
S.M.A.R.T. exercise and weight loss guidelines, 45, 46
smoking, 87, 95
sodium, 11, 21, 22, 33
statins, 76
steroids, 62, 82
stomach, 3
strength training, 43, 47
stress, 4, 61
reduction, 44

stress hormones, 4
stress test, 50
stroke, 1, 12, 15, 20, 76, 87–89
symptoms, 88
sugar
   see blood sugars, glucose
sulfonylureas, 66, 67
   side effects, 67
support group, 2
Surgeon General's Report on Physical Activity and Health, 48
symptoms of diabetes, 5, 6
syndrome x, 9
synthetic amylin hormone, 70
   side effects, 70
systolic blood pressure, 11

T

test strips, 55
testing sites for glucose meters, 56
testosterone replacement, 84
tests for type 2 diabetes, 6–9
thiazolidinediones (TZDs), 67
   side effects, 67

thrombosis, 88
toxemia, 93
trans fats, 21
triglycerides, 9, 11, 87
two-hour postprandial blood sugar level, 57
type 1 diabetes, 6
type 2 diabetes, 6
   complications, 78–96
   defining, 1–14
   managing, 13
   reversing, 12, 13
   symptoms, 5, 6
   testing, 6–9
types, 6

U

ulcers, 91, 95
unsaturated fats, 19
urinary tract, 81, 82, 83

V

vitamins, 34

W

warm-ups, 51
weakness, 63
weight control, 14–40, 79, 89, 94
weight gain, 4, 67, 68
weight loss, 5, 42, 70
weight loss tips, 37
white blood cells, 6

About the Authors

Rod Colvin, M.S., is a professional health writer and editor. In addition to editing dozens of books on consumer health, he is author of three other nonfiction books, including *Overcoming Prescription Drug Addiction*, Addicus Books, 2008.

A former journalist, Colvin holds a bachelor of arts degree from Washburn University in Topeka, Kansas, and a master of science degree in counseling psychology from Emporia State University in Emporia, Kansas.

James T. Lane, M.D., served as the medical editor for *Your Guide to Type 2 Diabetes.* Dr. Lane is the medical director of the Nebraska Medical Center Diabetes Center in Omaha, Nebraska. He is also an associate professor in the Department of Internal Medicine at the University of Nebraska Medical Center in Omaha.

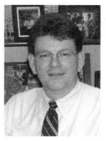

Dr. Lane earned his bachelor of arts degree and his medical degree from the University of Missouri in Kansas City, Missouri. He completed a residency in internal medicine at Rush-Presbyterian St. Luke's Medical Center, in Chicago, Illinois. He also completed fellowship training in endocrinology and metabolism at the University of Minnesota in Minneapolis.

As an active researcher, Dr. Lane's efforts have focused on the areas of diabetes-related complications, post-transplant diabetes, and the treatment of young adults with diabetes.

In 2001, Dr. Lane received the Top Teacher Award from the University of Nebraska Medical Center Department of Internal Medicine. In 2010, he received the Nebraska Medical Center Physician of Distinction for Medical Leadership Award for his work as a specialist in diabetes medicine.

Dr. Lane is a member of many professional organizations, including the American Diabetes Association, the Endocrine Society, the European Association for the Study of Diabetes, and the American Federation for Medical Research. He is also the author of numerous medical journal articles, abstracts, and chapters for textbooks.

A native of St. Louis, Dr. Lane currently makes his home in Omaha with his wife, Pascale, who is a pediatric nephrologist and a fellow diabetes researcher. They have two children, Jennifer and Tim.

Consumer Health Titles from Addicus Books
Visit our online catalog at www.AddicusBooks.com

After Mastectomy—Healing Physically and Emotionally . . $19.95
Bariatric Plastic Surgery $24.95
Body Contouring after Weight Loss $24.95
Cancers of the Mouth and Throat $14.95
Cataract Surgery $19.95
Colon & Rectal Cancer $14.95
Coronary Heart Disease $15.95
Countdown to Baby $19.95
The Courtin Concept—Six Keys to Great Skin at Any Age . $19.95
The Diabetes Handbook $19.95
Elder Care Made Easier $16.95
Exercising through Your Pregnancy $19.95
The Healing Touch $9.95
LASIK—A Guide to Laser Vision Correction $19.95
Living with P.C.O.S.—Polycystic Ovarian Syndrome . . . $19.95
Look Out Cancer Here I Come $19.95
Lung Cancer—A Guide to Treatment & Diagnosis $14.95
The Macular Degeneration Source Book $14.95
The New Fibromyalgia Remedy $19.95
The Non-Surgical Facelift Book—
    A Guide to Facial Rejuvenation Procedures $19.95
Overcoming Infertility $19.95
Overcoming Metabolic Syndrome $19.95
Overcoming Postpartum Depression and Anxiety $14.95
Overcoming Prescription Drug Addiction $19.95
Overcoming Urinary Incontinence $19.95
The New Fibromyalgia Remedy $19.95
A Patient's Guide to Dental Implants $14.95
Prostate Cancer $14.95
Sex and the Heart $19.95

To Order Books:

Visit us online at: www.addicusbooks.com

Call toll free: (800)-352-2873

For discounts on bulk purchases, call our Special Sales Dept. at (402) 330-7493